Curly Like Me

Curly Like Me

How to Grow Your Hair Healthy, Long, and Strong

Teri LaFlesh

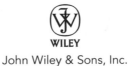

WILEY

John Wiley & Sons, Inc.

Copyright © 2010 by Teri LaFlesh. All rights reserved

Published by John Wiley & Sons, Inc., Hoboken, New Jersey
Published simultaneously in Canada

Illustrations © 2010 by Teri LaFlesh

Photo credits appear on page 267 and constitute an extension of the copyright page.

Design and composition by Forty-five Degree Design LLC

For general information about our other products and services, please contact our Customer Care Department within the United States at (800) 762-2974, outside the United States at (317) 572-3993 or fax (317) 572-4002.

Wiley also publishes its books in a variety of electronic formats. Some content that appears in print may not be available in electronic books. For more information about Wiley products, visit our web site at www.wiley.com.

Library of Congress Cataloging-in-Publication Data:

LaFlesh, Teri, date.
 Curly like me: how to grow your hair healthy, long, and strong / Teri LaFlesh.
  p. cm.
 Includes bibliographical references and index.
  ISBN 978-0-470-53642-1 (pbk.: alk. paper)
 1. Hairdressing—United States. 2. Hair—Care and hygiene—United States. 3. Racially mixed women—Health and hygiene—United States. 4. Beauty, Personal—Social aspects—United States. I. Title.
  TT972.L24 2010
  646.7'24—dc22

                                                                              2009031429

Printed in the United States of America

10 9 8 7 6 5 4 3 2 1

To my hair,
for all those years you only wanted to be yourself.

Contents

Acknowledgments

I am grateful and honored to have so many supportive people around me. I got superhuman help from some giving and patient people, without whom the book would still be a large stack of papers that continued to grow and hundreds of photos that continued to multiply.

I owe a gigantic thank-you to my agent, Emmanuelle Alspaugh, who proved she could move mountains and leap tall buildings. Because of her, this book is a reality. So many thanks to Arlene Robinson—this book's Fairy Godmother. Fate was kind the day she agreed to edit the first version of the manuscript. I'm grateful and stunned to be working with all of the wonderful people at Wiley and so happy to have found a home with them. Many large thank-yous to my editor, Christel Winkler, for her vision, support, and enthusiasm for this project—I'm elated to have this opportunity to work with her. Lisa Burstiner, the production editor, has turned my vision for the book into beautiful pages, and I am touched by the care and detail taken by her as well as copy editor Patricia Waldygo, who went over all my words to make them so much better. A big thanks to Betty Lowman for her enthusiasm and feedback and for putting me in touch with knowledgeable people; Photoshop master Hugh Macdonald, for walking me through much-needed techniques of preparing photos for printing; Kenneth Benson of Pegasus Type, for his meticulous help with InDesign when I was first starting out; Prema Qadir for her time and her honest feedback; and Daniel Bruce, for glancing over some last-minute additions.

More thanks than I can express to my mom for her constant support and being just fine with the alligator-loving little girl that I was, and to my dad for giving me his unique view of the world and showing me—literally and figuratively—that no door is locked until you try it. I am grateful to my stepmom, Ruth, for helping raise me and for all of her visits and inspiration through the years; my brother, Jeff, my childhood partner in crime (though probably not always by choice); Jeff's wife, Katrina; my sister, Chrystal; my mom's husband, Leon; and my dad's wife, Meredith, for sharing her curly-hair stories with me.

My life is so much richer for having my wonderful friends in it: Brewster, whom I have known longer than I haven't known; Deborah, for her kindnesses; Carrie, for being my SG; Miss Lena, for being a one-woman cheerleading squad; and, of course, Lena's wonderful parents, Bob and Essie, for their enthusiastic support of all of my creative projects, no matter how dubious—I am honored to have you in my life. Many thanks to Heidi Durrow for welcoming me to the table; to Amy and Monica for the dream of sand burrows; for all of the online support from Gillian, Maleka, Dione, my Farah, Benedicta, Vanessa, Aja, Jencie, Larene, Frances, Amber, and Lisa and for your suggestions, comments, advice, pictures, words, and friendship. I am indebted to all of the people who e-mailed me with their feedback, questions, photos, and suggestions: your encouragement and thoughtful questions made this book stronger.

This last giant thank-you I saved for my husband, Jon Crump. I am repeatedly stunned and honored by his love and perceptiveness that borders on psychic ability. He worked tirelessly on building the Web site and was an invaluable source of ideas, feedback, and support. He graciously let me use all of his cool software and even take over his computer. When things came down to the wire, he rolled up his sleeves and jumped in to help. I am continuously and happily surprised to have him in my life. Because of you, Jon, this book was possible.

Chapter One

My Hair History
How I Learned What Not to Do

used to think my hair was possessed. When I tried to comb or brush it, it turned into a frizzled netting. I used to feel like something was wrong with me because of my hair. Once I learned how to care for it, however, it became a cherished friend. I've found that with only a few simple changes in care, those same curls that once seemed possessed are now a feature I'm proud to have and are a joy to grow.

I arrived at this hard-won truth through years of fighting my hair and hating it, until I finally learned to love it as it is. By struggling against my natural hair, I turned what could have been sweet-natured curls into a broken beast. I wish I had known these things when I was younger; my teenage years would not have been so burningly awkward.

I wrote this book because I understand what it's like to go for years without knowing what to do with your hair and with little information available for guidance. I wanted others with very curly hair like mine to benefit from everything I learned during three decades of floundering. By reading this book, you won't have to struggle for answers anymore. *Curly Like Me* will serve as your "one-stop shopping" resource for very curly hair, where you can find information on your hair structure; what causes damage and how to prevent it; how to care for your curls; the best products, tools, and ingredients to use; and what happens when you use chemicals. I also include ideas for hairstyles that enhance your curls. This advice is streamlined and simple, because I want to show you how even the most uncoordinated person (such as myself) can easily enjoy her curls without employing an army of stylists. This book will tell you not only how to manage your curls, but also how to actually make them happy.

No prior experience is assumed, so a person who has never combed a curl in her life will be taught how to groom a head full of curls. This book is meant for people like me, who are not hairdressers and who don't have the time or energy to style their hair in elaborate, labor-intensive styles. *Curly Like Me* empowers you to take back the care of your own hair. It gives you the secrets to growing very long natural hair without feeling you must use costly treatments, products, or stylists.

The way to grow very long hair is simple: eliminate all sources of damage, and your hair will grow to its maximum length. The challenge, however, is that almost every conventional technique of caring for curly hair like ours causes damage. This book explains, step by step, how to care for your hair with almost zero damage. I do not promote trends, fads, or gimmicks. Even if some of what I say doesn't happen to be the most popular belief at the time, these techniques are the ones that work. I approach understanding your curls from many angles. First, I describe the highlights of my journey in learning how to take care of my hair. By repeatedly mangling my hair and after suffering through countless unfortunate hairstyles, I learned what didn't work for my curls. I also realized that by eliminating every product and procedure that would damage my hair, there was nothing to stop it from growing beautifully.

Next, *Curly Like Me* includes basic facts on the structure of hair and the bonds that hold the components of each individual hair together. Some of this information gets pretty technical, but it helps explain why your hair acts the way it does and what holds it together. This way, you'll learn what hurts your hair and how to avoid damaging it.

I'll describe each stage of caring for your hair, from washing and conditioning to combing extremely curly hair and to explaining how to grow it to its maximum length. I'll discuss which products work with your curls to make them much easier to groom. This will save you money you would spend on redundant products, as well as on those that don't work, and time you would waste on searching for magic products that don't exist. Although there are no miracle cures, and no product will substitute for good hair care and eliminating damage, you'll learn to use everyday products in unexpected ways to achieve amazing results. I'll tell you what ingredients to look for and to avoid and will give you product recommendations.

I'll also talk about what really happens when we apply chemicals to our hair. That section thoroughly explains the chemical bonds in our hair; it is at this molecular level where all the reactions take place when we permanently alter our curls. You don't have to read these chapters in order to use the techniques I'll teach you, though. This is a reference book on all aspects of tightly coiled hair, so feel free at first to skip around and use whatever chapters are helpful to you. Maybe after you find answers to your basic care questions, you'll become curious about the deeper structures within your curls.

I included photographs of hairstyles you can use to showcase your spiraling curls. These styles can be created quickly and easily, and you'll find instructions and illustrations for how to proceed. Most of these styles took only a few minutes each to achieve. There was no stylist standing by to make sure every strand was in place. I didn't use gel, hairspray, or styling tools of any sort (except my hands). I created each style myself, glanced in the mirror once when I was finished, sometimes made an adjustment or two, and took the picture with a timer.

Your curls might be a bit tighter or looser than mine, but the tips in this book will work if your hair is truly curly. Although you might need to modify my advice to suit your own unique curls, these ideas are a great starting point to help you understand how to work with your hair. None of these techniques will damage any type of hair but, rather, will help you enhance your curls rather than squish them down, hide them, alter them, or hurt them. Knowing how to care for your hair is much like opening a combination lock. Not only do you need to know all of the numbers and in what order they appear; you also need to be aware of which number to spin twice. Growing long, healthy curls is a similar process. You need to know all the techniques to grow your hair long and also figure out how they fit together. The lock won't open if you don't know which number has to go around twice, and growing healthy hair is much the same. You could be doing everything else right, but if you're still damaging your hair with one aspect of your regimen, it won't grow.

My Hair History

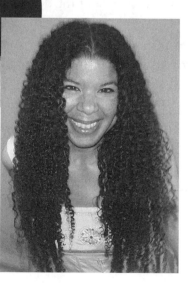

Before:
My chemically
damaged hair

and after:
my natural curls

I learned the hard way how to take care of my hair. Every useful technique I discovered was despite my own thick-headedness. Apparently, I'm one of those people who must try what doesn't work before she can find what does. I threw myself into each new attempt to change my hair and ended up with even worse hair damage than before I'd started. Only after I had tried everything to change what I was born with and had seen it fail did I finally stop running from my curls. I decided to face them, accept what I had, and make peace with them, and that was when everything changed. Following are the highlights of my journey.

Ever since I can remember, I wanted long mermaid hair—hair that flowed down my back, locks that I could toss dramatically over my shoulders. When I was a child, I stared at girls with hair longer than mine and tried to figure out how they got theirs to grow that way. It has taken me more than thirty years to learn how to have long hair falling down my back in a riot of spirals. Every lesson I learned, unfortunately, was at the expense of my hair. I was able to keep learning only because my curls kept growing back to give me one more chance to get it right.

Relaxed

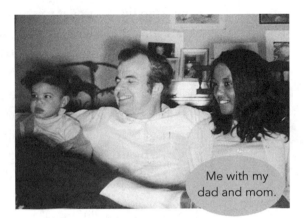

Me with my dad and mom.

I came by my curls by being black and white, and when I was a child—up until about fourth grade—Momsey, my black grandmother on my mom's side, did my hair. Each night she spent an hour combing, smoothing in French Perm hairdressing, and sectioning my hair into about twenty little balls over my head. Every few months my hair was relaxed; every few weeks it was washed. My straight hair strained to reach partway down my back. Momsey alone seemed to have the magic touch. My relaxed hair was a fragile creature, and we all seemed to tiptoe around it.

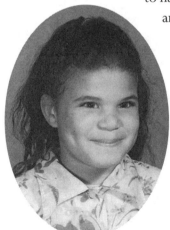

My third-grade school picture. My hair was a fragile thing, and lots of time and energy went into its maintenance.

I now think that because Momsey had been able to get my hair past my shoulders when I was a child, I spent the next twenty years trying to re-create what she had done (without success), instead of starting from scratch. Only after nothing worked for me did I try to do it my own way, without chemicals.

I spent my childhood summers in California with my dad, who is white. He and I were baffled by my hair, and he handled it the only way he knew how, which was to wash it with basic shampoo, not use any conditioner or moisturizer, blow it dry, brush it every day, and put it into two gigantic ponytail puffs with rubber bands. Because my hair had been relaxed during the school year, we could at least get a comb through it, if we were determined enough. Each year my hair got shorter.

My mom, distressed that my hair kept getting shorter instead of longer, took me to a hairdresser when I was eleven to see whether a professional could stop the damage. I was taken to a back room where, inexplicably, my hair was cut very short and I was given a Jheri curl. The curl was put on top of the relaxer that had been applied to my natural curls. I cried when I looked in the mirror and saw all my hair gone. It would take me more than eighteen years to figure out how to get it long again.

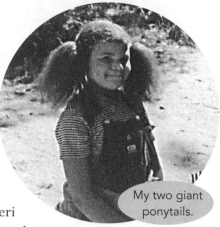

My two giant ponytails.

Over the summer I visited my dad, who saw the greasy activator I'd brought with me, and requested that I not use it. As the summer progressed, the dried-out Jheri curl became further damaged from the harsh shampoos, no conditioning rinses or any other moisturizers, and daily dry brushing. I just brushed my hair and tried to pat it into a round shape as best I could. Had I understood then that that tormented chemical mess wasn't what my natural hair was really like, I would never have

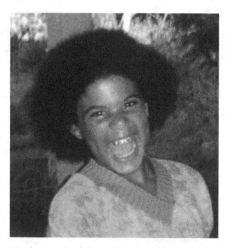

By the end of the summer, my triple-damaged hair (Jheri curl that was applied over the relaxer that was initially used on my curls, plus daily dry brushing) grew larger and stiffer.

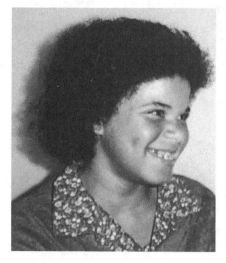

This shows the crunchy texture of the dried-out Jheri curl.

gone through all of the ensuing battles with chemicals trying to avoid the hair I experienced that summer.

My grandmother on my father's side wanted to try to help me by styling my hair herself after hearing (probably for the thousandth time) my frustrated complaints about not knowing what to do with it. She had two daughters of her own, and she assured me that she knew how to do hair. One day during a summer visit, she worked earnestly to style my hair with her curling iron. My hair's consistency was like that of warm plastic. After that, my grandmother didn't bring up the subject of hair again. At the end of the summer, when I returned to my mom's house, my hair was immediately relaxed, and would continue to have chemicals in it for the next twenty years.

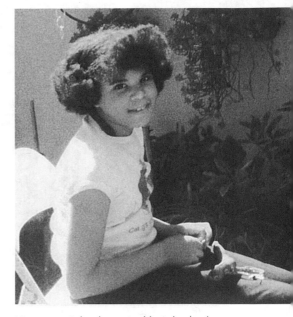

How my triple-damaged hair looked after styling with a curling iron.

In my early teens, I moved to California during the school months and was suddenly left alone with my hair full time. I put relaxer on it to tame the curls and always ended up burning myself. My clumsy application of the chemicals left second-degree burns and scabs behind my ears for weeks. My hair was so damaged, it broke off at my shoulders, and it was still unmanageable. After I washed my hair, my arms ached from trying to get a comb through it. I spent hours trying to comb it, and still it was a fuzzy nest. I often ended up with the comb tangled in my hair at some point during the process. Frantic, I mentally yelled at my hair and usually ended up in tears before I was finished combing and setting it. Suffering from its own torment, my hair continued to arc off my head as if my scalp were electrified.

It was just that hair and me alone together, and I tried everything I could think of to make it presentable. I wrangled curlers and rollers into it each night. Then I couldn't sleep because they jabbed my head all over, and I became an insomniac. In the morning, my hair would still be half-wet in the back and would fuzz when I took out the curlers. I looked for

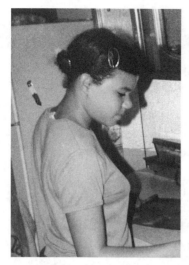

The only way I could wear my relaxed hair was by strapping it down as tightly as possible.

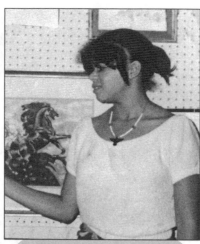

It was so stiff that it stuck up in the air when I wore it in ponytails or braids. This is me at a very crabby moment.

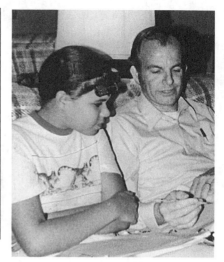

Me, my dad, and my curlers. I put my hair in curlers at night because I couldn't think of anything else to do with it.

a magic shampoo, conditioner, treatment, or ingredient to make it act like everyone else's naturally straight hair, then I searched for a miraculous hairdressing to weigh it down and make it grow, as they all promised to do. But all that these potions and lotions left behind were grease stains on everything my hair came in contact with. I startled people whenever I wore a white T-shirt to school. My back and shoulders were always covered in broken hair bits, as if I'd gotten caught in a violent hair-snipping storm.

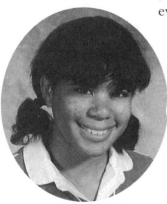

This was my usual hairstyle during most of high school.

When I put my hair into a braid, I needed a ponytail holder made of onyx to fasten it. Onyx was the only thing heavy enough to weigh down the braid. Without it, my braid stuck out like an antenna, as if intently listening to something far up in the sky.

I went to an all-white school (well, sometimes there was one other person of color in the entire school), and I lived with my all-straight-haired white side of the family. Heck, even my brother had wavy hair. People around me could easily run combs through their hair like it was no big deal. Their combs would emerge from the ends of their untangled hair, which then flowed back into place as if nothing had happened. They shrugged off rain or wind. Their hair was shiny and long, and they could toss it in the wind. They could braid it casually, and the braids lay where they put them. My hair seemed to enjoy singling me out and making sure I never forgot I was different. I hated my hair, so I punished it as severely as I felt punished by it.

Salons

When I was fifteen, my dad took me to a salon to get my hair professionally relaxed, to see whether that might work better for me than doing it myself. The chemicals seared my scalp—the hairdresser left them on for the full amount of time. Then she put me in tight rollers under a hot hood dryer. She burned my forehead when she used the curling iron on my bangs, and teased my hair in a bouffant hairdo. Afterward, my hair was crunchy and my scalp ached, as if my hair had been put on way too tight. My head glowed with heat for days, and I knew that this wasn't the solution I wanted either. So I kept walking around with my shirts covered in broken hair bits while I cast about for a better way.

Every couple of years I took a pair of household scissors and, in frustration, hacked off my hair down to a few inches. Just after I cut it all off in the summer before eleventh grade, I dyed my hair bright orange and decided something had to be done.

Locks

In twelfth grade I tried dreadlocks. I thought locks were exotic and lovely and maybe my ticket to long, flowing hair. That I had no idea how to grow them didn't slow me down. I thought my hair would just naturally separate and lock on its own if I simply stopped combing it for long enough. Instead, after a few months of not being combed, my hair turned into a solid mat on my head. I tore it apart in sections and then cut out chunks to form the individual locks.

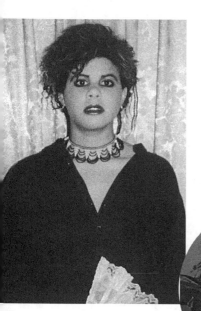

After I had separated my mats into individual locks, I waited impatiently for my hair to finally grow. The individual locks stuck straight out all over my head like the spines of a sea urchin, refusing to lie flat. I sewed glass beads onto each lock to weigh it down. Every few months I measured one of them. In a year, they hadn't grown. Near the end of twelfth grade, I finally chopped them off with kitchen scissors and was back to short hair again. (I now know that my hair actually *was* growing, but because it was also still locking and tightening at the same time, its growth and the process of locking probably just evened each other out.)

Mistakenly thinking that the hair I'd experienced after the Jheri curl *was* what my natural hair was like, I decided to relax my hair again. To have those curls with no restraint seemed so out of the question, I didn't even consider it.

Pre-dreads:
I was cultivating my unimat. Not knowing how to start locks, I rubbed my hair with a towel. Of course, this just made my hair turn into one large mat.

My hair was usually orange or red at this time.

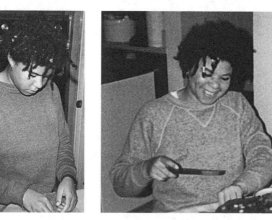

Here I am with locks that never grew and the beads sewn in to keep them weighed down (you can see the bands of beads as white in my hair in these photos).

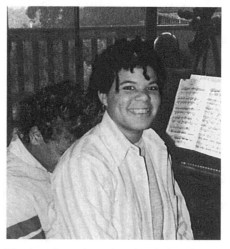

My dreads, with my brother behind me.

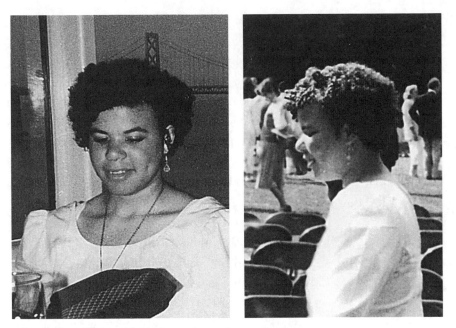

I'd cut off my locks with kitchen scissors by graduation.

The Fateful Relaxer

Although it had been more than a year since I'd last used a perm, I felt like I still remembered the drill when I brought it home from the store. It was early summer at my mom's house in Kentucky. I opened the larger jar in the relaxer kit, nonchalantly slathered it on my head, and waited the given amount of time. When I rinsed my hair, I was annoyed to see that nothing had happened. I checked the instructions and saw, too late, that I should have mixed the ingredients. I promptly bought another relaxer kit to do it right this time.

The second time around, everything seemed fine until I went to rinse. The relaxer wouldn't come out. With the addition of water, my hair had turned into a gooey paste. I rinsed and shampooed repeatedly, growing more panicked each time. As the goo reluctantly gave way, my hair came out with it—in handfuls that filled the sink basin. When my hair was dry, what was left of it crunched like a dead leaf. The next day, I put on a hat and went shopping for weaves.

Weaves

In search of the elusive mermaid hair, I walked into a weave shop for the first time. All my life I had wanted long, thick hair to throw dramatically back over my shoulders, and suddenly there was an entire wall filled with just such hair in every beautiful color and texture. And any of them could be mine. I started out with dark honey-brown wefts in a straightened texture; these seemed to match the color of my damaged hair. After a little instruction from the man behind the counter, I was wearing my new weave.

I loved it. At last, I instantly had the hair I'd dreamed of, flowing past my shoulders. Finally, I could pull it back in a long ponytail or braid, and it hung the way I had always imagined hair should. It didn't matter about the rain or the wind or the humidity. I felt like a movie star and immediately became addicted to weaves. Every couple of weeks I visited the shop again to try a new length or texture. When I took my new hair home on the bus, I'd open the bag it was in and smell that new hair smell wafting faintly from inside its paper cocoon.

Me looking artsy—but not happy—in my bulky weave.

There were some significant drawbacks to the weaves, however. The foremost was that they were easy to see. The weft was always a challenge to hide near the hairline. You could see that strip of fabric the hair was sewn into, so a big part of doing my hair was thinking of ways to hide it. My own hair was too short and crunchy to do a good job of covering it, so I ended up wearing a scarf around my head most of the time to hide where the weave started.

The weaves were also very hard to take down and comb, and they always seemed to be shedding. I glued the hair to the weft to keep it from coming out, but that made it lumpier on my head. Beneath my weave lurked a broken mess, but I prized the feel of long and thick hair too much to think about what was really going on under the facade.

My biggest fear with weaves was of detection. I was a fake. It was not my own hair, and I was always afraid people could tell—which I'm sure they could. I kept imagining, for example, a cute guy putting his hand in my hair, unexpectedly contacting the tumorlike lumps of the wefts and snatching his hand away in horror and betrayal. I was determined to have glamorous hair that was less detectable. This was the reason I began to wear extensions.

Extensions

I bought bags of loose hair and tried to figure out how to put it in. At the time I couldn't find any literature on how to do it, but stuff like that doesn't seem to stop me. I experimented with how to get the additional hair to stay in my existing hair. One of my earlier attempts was to clip the loose ends of the extension hair to the beginning of my hair and simply start braiding the two together. After putting in a few dozen braids, the loose hairs of the extension poked into my scalp and itched to the point that I had to take them out. A friend who had them finally showed me how her hairdresser had put them in. I tried using nylon hair, but it looked like doll hair. Besides, it would frizzle in the blast of heat from an opened oven if I was standing too close and not paying attention.

To save the hundreds to thousands of dollars it would have cost to have my hair done by people who knew what they were doing, I did my hair on my own. It took weeks of working on it for three or four hours a night until I got all of the braids in. By the time I finished the back, it was time to redo the front. I grew more reluctant to tackle combing out each braid, because my hair was locking into the extensions. I procrastinated for nearly a year, until the fear of my hair bonding to the braids motivated me to take them out.

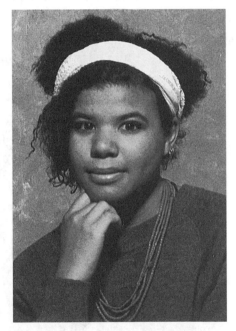

This is what my hair looked like when I took out the weaves. It was just starting to grow in after the Fateful Relaxer. At night I slept in a bandanna to try to smash down my hair.

I spent twenty-four hours tearing out the extensions, which left me with a head full of hundreds of cylindrical mats, all netted together. The following day it took me eight hours to comb these appendages out. When I was finished, I ended up with a fuzz ball the size of a Pomeranian. I decided that I didn't have enough discipline to keep up with this style, so again it was time to look for an alternative that worked for me.

Texturizing

I went back to the chemicals, but this time I tried texturizing: leaving the relaxer on for a shorter amount of time, just to loosen the curl. I'd worn my hair this way for a while in high school, and I recalled that it had required the least amount of maintenance of all my 'dos. I texturized for several years. Although I liked the curls, they were highly damaged, frizzed easily, and were unpredictable. With high humidity or too much wind, they turned into a big halo of fuzz (not that there's anything wrong with a halo of fuzz; I didn't like feeling trapped into only one look, and at the time, I desperately wanted my hair to act more like the straighter hair of those around me). I used gel and mousse in my attempt to define and

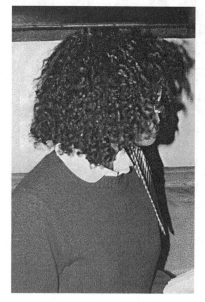
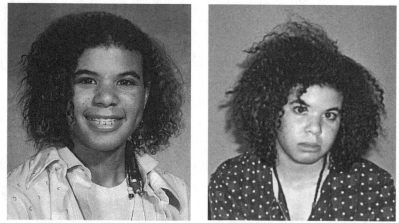

Texturized through the years: in high school, in eleventh grade (in the middle picture, I hacked off the front of my hair down to half an inch), and in young adulthood. My face expresses how my chemically texturized hair must have been feeling.

emphasize the curls and prevent the frizz, but these products made them tight and stiff, like lots of little crunchy strings.

Once, while experimenting with texturizing in high school, I ended up with one side of my hair straight, the other side curly. I couldn't afford more perm at the time, so every morning I intently scrunched up the straight side and tried to flatten out the curly side so that they matched. It didn't work. My straight/curly head fascinated yet puzzled my friends in my all-naturally-straight-haired school, who were especially struck by the seam at the back of my head where the two types of hair met.

Bit o' Everything

There were a couple years when I had multiple styles going on at once. I had lots of new growth, texturized hair, relaxed hair, and even a few braided extensions thrown in for good measure.

During all of my experiments, what concerned me the most was that my hair would not grow. It shied away from my shoulders as if they were dangerous. I knew better than to let my hair blow in

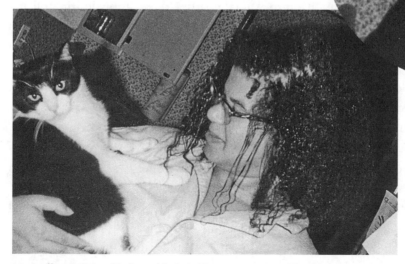

You can see my extensions in this photo. I put in only a few of them, just in the front, for some reason. I think I liked hair hanging in my face at that time.

My puffy texturized/relaxed hair (with my angry cat, Elmer).

the wind, and there was nothing to swing over my shoulders. If texturizing had been the right option for my hair, I decided, it would thrive and grow to its maximum length, not continue to break off. Because my hair was still short, it meant that texturizing wasn't the answer.

This realization became my turning point: I felt as if I'd tried everything, and nothing had worked. So, if everything I tried didn't work, what about trying nothing?

I'd once read a magazine article that said the less you do to your hair, the healthier it will be. Where did that leave me? It's easy for the author to say that, I thought resentfully. I have to straighten my big mess of hair. My hair was so out of control *with* straightening, I couldn't even imagine what horrors would erupt without it. Then one day in a bookstore while searching for answers, I happened upon *Good Hair: For Colored Girls Who've Considered Weaves When the Chemicals Became Too Ruff* by Lonnice Brittenum Bonner. This brave author had grown out her relaxer and had lived to tell about it. Reading about her experience, I felt that if she could do it, then I had no excuse for not trying.

Growing It Out, Setting It Free

Too chicken to cut off all of my hair, I chose to grow the chemicals out instead. Yet growing it out was much harder than simply cutting off the chemicals and starting fresh. For the first few months, my hair matted where the two types of hair met, and my comb halted at the divide and didn't want to budge. Not only did my comb get stuck in the mat, the mat was too close to my scalp for me to keep it from being pulled and hurting. I hoped beyond hope that the mat was simply the place where the two textures of hair joined, not a waking monster slowly emerging from my scalp. I set my hair in two stranded twists to hide the different textures.

Over the next four months or so, to my relief, the mat line inched down my head. I realized that the comb was gliding through the new growth but halting at the boundary where the chemicals had been applied to my hair. This was a revelation and my first glimmer of hope. It meant that my new growth wasn't causing the trouble after all; it was the chemically damaged hair.

When It Clicked

After eight months, I noticed something amazing. One night I lifted up the hair behind my ear and looked at the new growth coming in. There, for the first time, I saw my *real* hair. It was in a perfectly formed S-pattern that seemed as unique as my own fingerprint. The new growth was slippery, smoother than I'd ever felt my hair to be. The texture of my hair within that short length was firm and confident. It shone like obsidian. Realizing that this beautiful hair was waiting for me beneath the crunchy chemical hair, I couldn't stand to put it off any longer. I cut all of the old, broken, chemically damaged hair off my head. That stuff wasn't really my hair anyway.

For the first time in my life I saw what my real hair looked like. Confident and glossy, it was radically different from the chemically destroyed hair that had clung to the bottom of it.

Those new curls were vibrant and so different from the damaged mess I'd mistakenly thought was my hair all my life. Now that the damage was gone, my entire head of hair felt different from how it ever had before. It was soft and shiny, even directly after shampooing. The curls were firm and confident. I'd never experienced this creature before, and I became suddenly and fiercely protective of these fresh curls unfurling from my head like new fronds on a fern. If I could figure out a way to go without damaging them, I speculated, then my hair could potentially grow to its maximum length. Knowing that hair grows an average of six inches a year, I held a yardstick to the area behind my ear to see where the lengths would fall. How long would two years of growth be? Three years? Six years of unbroken growth? The yardstick reached past my stomach. Could my hair really grow that long? And with curls? That last question worried me. All of the literature I'd read said that really curly hair couldn't grow long, because weakness was built into every twist and turn in every strand of hair. This implied that my curly hair by its nature was flawed, destined to break before it even made it

What my new growth looked like the first time I saw it, gleaming against my broken, chemically treated hair.

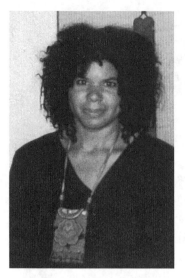

My hair when most of the chemicals were first cut off. As my chemical-free hair was growing, I still wasn't sure what to do with it. My curls lost their definition when the weather was humid.

out of the gate. I examined the strands of my new curls. They looked like little springs, but the strands were continuous. To me, they didn't seem flawed or dented at every twist. So, I wondered, maybe it was the damage from trying to force these twists and turns to do something they weren't meant to do that had hurt them, and not something inherent in their structure?

Well, I *was* doing something radically different with my hair this time. I hoped I had figured out the missing puzzle piece I'd been looking for all along. Since that day when I first saw my real hair, I never straightened it again, and it grew year by year. The first couple of years of growth produced a crown of thick, glossy curls instead of the crunchy hair I'd gotten used to. It just kept growing longer and longer: to my shoulders, passing my shoulders, and down my back. All the while, I kept experimenting with how best to comb and style it, to make the most of its coils, and above all, to never harm it again.

Conditioning and Separating

During this time, my hair and I were still getting to know each other. In rain or humid weather, my hair still blew up like a threatened puffer fish as the curls lost definition and expanded. They were still generally unpredictable, and I wanted to find a way to define those lovely

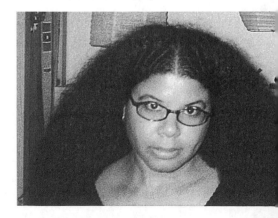

Although my hair was longer than it had ever been, it was still poufy and unpredictable. I searched for how to define my curls. My mother called lots of tiny waves erupting from a person's head a "porridge head," though I'm not sure why. I have a slicked-back porridge head here. In fact, I had lots of porridge action going on whenever it was humid.

new curls I had. Yet I now felt that my hair was my friend, and I wanted to work with it to make us as happy together as possible.

With my hair now reaching to the small of my back when wet, I discovered a technique that made all the difference: leaving the conditioner in and then separating my hair into individual curls. Separating them freed my curls to do their own thing; it defined each one, instead of my combing the curl until it merged into its neighbors. With each curl defined and soothed with conditioner, I could finally wear my hair in a long ponytail that hung heavy against my back. Humidity no longer mattered, nor did wind or rain. This, it turned out, was the final puzzle piece I'd been missing.

Now

I no longer spend hours frustrated and trying to "fix" my hair and then many more hours attempting to undo whatever terrible thing I've done to "fix" it in the first place. At night, I simply twist it into a bun or a braid, and in the morning I take it down and style it in a couple of minutes. After a weekly combing, the rest of the week I might spend one to ten minutes a day on it, at the most. I can have my hair pinned up, and whenever I feel like it, I can unpin it and it falls down over my shoulders. My curls are good-natured—they let me do what I want with them as long as I don't hurt them anymore, which seems to work out well for both of us.

Afros are fiercely beautiful. What I had when I was eleven, however, was not my natural hair. It was a chemically induced mess. The triple whammy of the relaxer, the Jheri curl over it, and no conditioner or moisturizer, plus the daily dry brushing left it stiff, crunchy, and brutalized. The unfortunate thing was, being a child, I didn't realize that that hair wasn't really my hair. I had no idea of the damage those chemical treatments did to it. I mistakenly thought that the way my hair felt, looked, and acted was what my hair was like when it was worn naturally curly. Because of this belief, it took me nearly twenty years to discover that that hair was not my real hair. And really, if you think about it, the way I have my hair now is simply a curly natural hair that's grown down to my hips.

As my hair has grown longer, tight spirals at the end of each curl act like counterweights that pull the rest of the curl down. After twelve years of chemical-free growth, my hair is down to my hips. I use few products on my hair: shampoo, a couple of conditioners for variety, and occasionally a bit of olive or coconut oil on my ends in the driest days of winter. I no longer spend hundreds of dollars and frustrated hours in stores searching for some magic potion that will fix my hair. I know that product doesn't exist. Preventing damage and knowing how to treat my curls are the true magic formula and the only one that works.

Now I realize that for decades, I had tried to tame my curls into obedience by forcing them to conform to the kind of hair that others had. I treated my curls as if they weren't good enough in their natural state. Yet after all I had done to them, they couldn't be crushed. Patiently, they kept growing back, each new head of hair giving me yet one more chance to do better.

As I have found in life, sometimes the truth turns out not to be what I first thought I wanted. But whenever I accept it, embrace it, and learn to

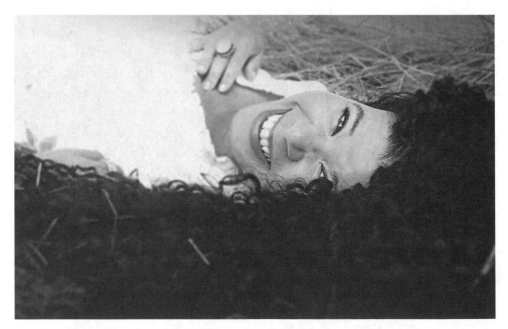

I found that when I made peace with my hair, I made peace with myself.

celebrate the unique opportunity that the truth gives me to grow and to learn, I become richer for having done so. So it is with my hair. The hair I once felt so ashamed of has now become my best feature. You see, as it turns out, I have been given the gift of tightly spiraled hair that relatively few people have.

Your curls are wonderful and special. In the following pages, I'll tell you what I've discovered through decades of struggle and research, and I'll give you all of the keys I've found to help you make *your* beautiful curls naturally long, defined, and happy.

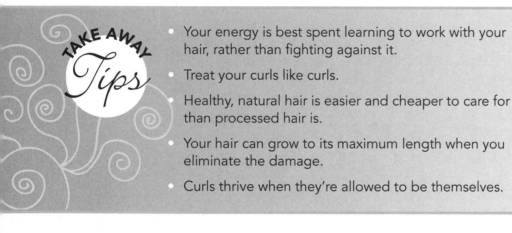

TAKE AWAY Tips

- Your energy is best spent learning to work with your hair, rather than fighting against it.

- Treat your curls like curls.

- Healthy, natural hair is easier and cheaper to care for than processed hair is.

- Your hair can grow to its maximum length when you eliminate the damage.

- Curls thrive when they're allowed to be themselves.

Chapter Two

Get to Know Your Curls
Their Structure and Vulnerabilities

Whenever I pass a tree, my hair grabs onto the bark. It catches on the rough grain in wood furniture and wraps around buttons, sequins, and other people's watches. It's so curly, a brush doesn't go through it. I get my comb tangled in it every time I comb it. I once had rice poured on my head, and my hair was still raining rice three days later, even after washing and combing.

What makes our hair so curly? What goes on inside those tendrils that makes them so perfect for grabbing? We are caught in the paradox of having hair so thick and rebellious that a comb won't go through it when it's dry, but so fragile it breaks if treated harshly. Because it's as

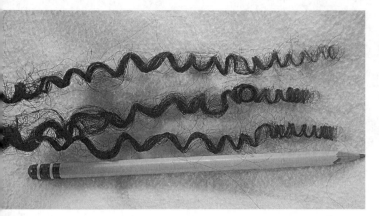

My spirals are the diameter of a pencil, and they are perfectly made for catching and holding onto things. They are the exact shape that nature has given plants when they need an appendage to grab onto things for support, like the tendrils of pea plants and morning glory vines.

My hair turns into netting when it's combed dry.

fine as gossamer, when we comb it while dry, our hair seems to turn into netting.

This chapter burrows deep into the structure of your curls. If you understand what makes your hair the way it is, you'll be better equipped to make decisions to protect it. It is within this hidden world that the answers to your hair reside.

Hair Thickness

Our curly hair is usually very fine, which is one reason we have some of the challenges we do. You see, hair comes in a range of thicknesses, from wiry to fine, depending on the diameter of each hair. Coarse or wiry hair might feel harder to the touch and sleeker, because each strand is much thicker than fine or medium hair. This hair can be resistant to styling. Since the individual strands are thicker, they are much stronger. Medium hair is softer than coarse hair because each hair has a smaller diameter than coarser hair does. Fine hair tends to feel soft and downy to the touch. The strands have a small diameter, so although there might be lots of hair, each individual strand is delicate. Fine hair often lacks the medulla, the inner core that other hair types have. One person can have a mixture of hair thicknesses.

Hair can also feel thicker on the head depending on how many actual strands there are, as well as on the amount of curl each strand has. Because a curl takes up more space than a strand of straighter hair, curly hair feels thick, although each individual strand might be gossamer thin. This explains why your hair might seem stubborn and tough. It's really just thousands of delicate, thin, fluffy strands, the masses of them making your hair seem as though it can take almost anything. Think of your hair more as a frightened, fluffed-up kitten. It might seem big and tough, but it's actually delicate and easily hurt.

This book will focus mainly on fine to medium hair, because this is the hair I learned how to handle and the hair most of us of African descent have. In addition, African American hair tends to be finer than other racial hair types, up to 84 percent thinner than the thickest Asian hair. Had my hair been coarse, it most likely would not have been as devastated by the perms I used. Because my hair is soft and fine, however, the chemicals I once used ravaged it, destroying the strands so that they broke instead of grew.

It's crucial to understand how the diameter of your hair determines what kind of treatment it can handle. The diameter controls how your hair reacts to damage, so it's directly related to how long your hair can grow under various circumstances. Thicker strands of hair can withstand more damage than fine hairs can. This is similar to how a thick tree trunk can survive a few chops with an ax that would fell a thin sapling. People with thicker strands of hair can do more damaging things to it and still grow it pretty long. True, it might have thousands of split ends and may look dull, and I'm not saying it's okay to damage any hair, but thick hair doesn't fall apart. Those of us with thinner strands of hair could do the exact same thing to our hair, but ours *would* fall apart.

For example, my mom was able to relax her hair and grow it halfway down her back. Seeing that she could still have long hair, even though it was relaxed, made me think I should be able to do the same thing. What

I didn't realize is that my mom has thicker strands of hair than I do. Therefore, my hair simply fell apart when I applied the same chemicals to mine that she applied to hers. So, it's true that some people will be able to relax or perm their hair, and it might still grow long. Mine will not. If the individual strands of your hair are thin, you might not have had any luck with perms, either. This is why my hair grew only when I stopped using chemicals on it.

Hair Phases: How Much of Your Hair Is Growing at Any One Time?

Hair is dynamic. All of the hair on your head is at one of three stages: growing, resting, or packing up and leaving. At any given time, as long as you're in good health, most of your hair is growing. Each hair grows for about two to seven years, and nearly 90 percent of your hair will be in this growth stage. Your health and your genes determine how much time your hair spends growing. The more time each hair has to grow, the longer your hair will be. Most people have hair that can grow long enough to reach down to the middle of their backs. They just don't realize it. Hair often doesn't *seem* to grow when it's being damaged and breaking off at the same rate (or worse, faster than) it grows. While a few people can grow hair long enough to step on, there are others who have hair that's genetically programmed to reach only a little past their shoulders before each hair's life span ends.

During the resting stage, your hair prepares for the end of its time on your scalp. Only about 12 percent of your hair is in this holding pattern at a time. After three to eight weeks of resting, your hair has said its good-byes and is now ready to go. After a hair falls out, the follicle rests for about twelve to sixteen weeks before building another hair and starting the process all over again. Each follicle is capable of about twenty of these cycles before it runs out of steam and stops producing. We shed about 100 to 150 hairs a day (although in pregnancy, that number might drop until a woman is shedding only 15 to 20 hairs a day). Provided that you're in good health, this equals about 700 to nearly 1,050 hairs lost a week. This means that if you comb your hair once a week, there will be a mat the size of a tiny animal left in your comb. This is totally normal.

It's important to know the average life span of a hair, because you need a marker to determine when your (or someone else's) hair is healthy enough to have most likely reached its maximum length. This means it's grown its entire life with so little damage that it didn't break off before it could grow as long as it was genetically programmed to. Hair that has grown to an average maximum length lives about six years (for some people it's much less time, and for some it's much more). This is about thirty-six inches, or lower-back length, depending on how fast it grows. If you can't get your hair to grow to its maximum length (shorter than your lower back when gently stretched), it means that in some way your hair is still being damaged.

The Basic Structure of Your Curls

Your hair is made up of layers, like a tree. And similar to the tree's bark, your hair's protective outer layer, the cuticle, is composed of multiple overlapping scales. This layer covers and protects the fragile core within it: the cortex. Under the cortex, especially in people who have coarser hair, is a central air-filled core called the medulla. The thickness of the medulla is similar to the way thicker trees have more rings that add to the diameter of their trunks than thinner trees have.

The Cuticle

Your cuticle layer holds each of your hairs together and protects it. When the cuticle is destroyed, the center of each hair quickly follows. Every strand of your hair is covered five to ten shingles deep, much like the shingles of a roof (if that roof happened to have five to ten layers of shingles, that is). The shingles of the cuticle look like transparent, overlapping scales. These overlapping layers grow facing down, which is why it feels so unpleasant to run your hand up your hair. You're going against all of those millions of microscopic scales that cover all the strands of your hair.

When these scales are intact and lying against one another, your hair looks shiny. It shines because the cuticles reflect light like a smooth sheet of glass. When the cuticle is damaged by rough towel drying, shampooing, perming, frequent or rough brushing, backcombing, or burning with flatirons, the scales are roughed up and torn off. And just like glass that has been ground down, scratched, and chipped, the cuticle becomes dull and no longer shines.

The Cortex

The cuticle shields the fragile center of each hair: the cortex. The cortex is like your hair's database. It holds the very characteristics that make your hair look and behave the way it does. When your cuticle is destroyed, the cortex (the spongy center) is left exposed and defenseless. Once the cuticle is gone, the cortex succumbs easily to destruction. After damage of any kind is done, it's permanent until the damaged part is cut off or replaced by fresh new hair. Conditioners can coat the cuticles to make them more slippery, but once the cuticles are damaged, they can't ever be repaired.

The cortex gives your hair its personality, because it determines the color, elasticity, and curl of your hair. Every cortex is composed of coiled keratin fibers twisted together like thin lengths of rope, which are then bundled to make thicker lengths of fiber. Lots of these fibers are finally bundled together to compose the cortex. The cortex also houses a mixture of pigment granules, and these give your strands their own unique color.

The Medulla

The very center of your hair strand might contain a medulla. The medulla is often present only in people with coarser hair, and sometimes it doesn't even run the entire length of each hair. The medulla is mostly filled with air held in a honeycomb pattern of keratin. In the coats of many animals, this air-filled layer acts as insulation to keep them warm. It's believed that the medulla's presence in our hair might be a remnant from the time when we were also covered with hair.

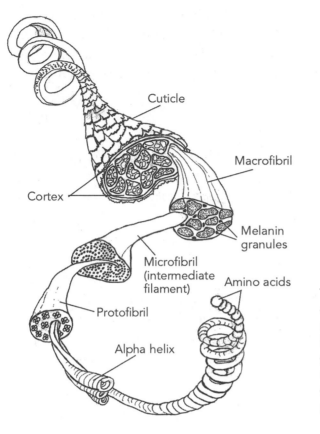

Cuticle

Macrofibril

Cortex

Melanin granules

Microfibril (intermediate filament)

Amino acids

Protofibril

Alpha helix

This is a cross-section of what one of our very curly hairs might look like. Because our hair tends to be very fine, it generally doesn't have a medulla (the hollow air-filled core that is sometimes present in coarser hairs).

I wish I'd known much sooner what was really preventing me from growing long hair. Because I had no idea about the structure of my hair and how my thin strands of hair were affected by damage, I was always coming up with odd schemes to grow it. All the while, I didn't know that the chemicals I used on it had already fatally wounded my hair, and no product could bring it back to health.

The Ways Your Hair Is Damaged

The cuticle layers over the fragile cortex in each of your hairs to protect it. Without protection, the cortex quickly unravels, and your hair falls apart. Hair can't repair itself, so once it's damaged, there's no solution but for us to cut it off. To keep your hair healthy and to grow the longest hair possible, it's best to avoid hurting it in the first place. Unfortunately, there are many ways your hair can be damaged, such as sun exposure, rough handling, backcombing, heat styling, bleaching, and perming.

Sun Damage

When you leave your hair unprotected while under the sun, ultraviolet light can damage it, in the same way that bleach can. Sun exposure not only lightens your hair, it also weakens your hair and dries it out. Once hair is weakened, it splits open and breaks off.

Rough Handling

You can damage your hair in several ways by treating it roughly, such as by dry brushing, rough shampooing, rough towel drying, or wrapping a rubber band too tightly around it. Brushing hair frequently or roughly will wear out anyone's hair, but for our very curly strands, the damage can be intense. In *Don't Go Shopping for Hair-Care Products without Me*, Paula Begoun wrote, "Without question, brushing is one of the most damaging things you do to your hair. . . . Every time you brush through your hair, the bristles or spikes chip away at the cuticle."

In addition, brushing through thick hair, especially when it's dry, requires a certain amount of force. It takes muscle to pull a brush through an expanded net of twists and curls. The force that you use wears away your cuticles and, worse, stretches your hair, weakening its fiber, often well past the breaking point.

Piling your hair on top of your head and rubbing shampoo vigorously into it or roughly grinding the towel into wet hair to dry it will not only rough up your cuticles, but is the express route to matting your hair. Putting hair bands on your hair too tightly will twist and rip the cuticles from your hair. Once the cuticle is gone, the cortex doesn't stand a chance.

It might not seem like such a big deal to roughly yank your comb through your hair this one time or to use scorching heat on your hair just this once. But we rarely ever do anything once in the life span of our hair.

If you tend to yank your comb through your hair when you comb it or rub the towel into it after washing it, you probably do it almost every time.

Now multiply this act by how often it happens during the life of each strand of hair. If your hair grows an average of, say, seven years, and you comb it roughly every week, this means that by the time your hair has reached maturity, it will have gone through 364 rough combings. Twice a week means 728 times. If you were to brush a piece of fabric roughly 364 to 728 times or more, it would wear away and look ragged very quickly. Keep this in mind for anything that you do to your hair. Whatever you do, your hair rarely has to endure it only one time (although there are some things so damaging that you only have to do them once to hurt your hair). It's usually the little things that don't seem so bad when you do them ("just this one time because I'm in a hurry") that add up. Due to this gradual damage, it will be nearly impossible for you to put your finger on why your hair looks dry and damaged or your ends broken and split. This process happens little by little, and you don't see it. Always keep this in mind, whatever you do to your hair or when you are deciding what to do to your hair: Multiply it by how many times it will happen in your hair's lifetime. If the procedure will destroy fabric, it will destroy your hair.

Backcombing

Combing your hair in the opposite direction of growth causes severe damage to your cuticles. In electron-microscope images of backcombed hair, the scales look like they've been rolled back up the hair shaft like a tube sock that has been rolled down a leg. Backcombing not only pulls off your cuticles, but also crams all the roughed-up hairs together in a matted pocket. As a result, vigorous combing and tugging are required to undo the bird's nest that was created this way.

Heat Damage

Your hair consists of 10 to 13 percent water, even when it's dry. When wet, it can absorb up to one-third of its weight in water. Water boils at 212 degrees Fahrenheit. Blow dryers and curling irons can reach temperatures of up to 392 degrees, flatirons can be nearly 450 degrees, and pressing combs can reach a whopping 500 degrees. What this means is that these hairstyling tools can boil the water inside your hair shaft. The steam from the boiling water expands inside your shaft and creates bubbles within your hair. Now, if that happens with the tiny bit of moisture that's inside dry hair, imagine what the high heat does to wet hair! Because your hair has absorbed a third of its weight in additional water, there is now more water to boil and burst within it. Your hair then breaks off all around these blisters.

In addition, the intense heat from hair pressing causes a sweeping loss of cuticles, resulting in hair fracture and loss. Flat ironing makes your hair feel smooth, but this is because the cuticles are often melted together, with the damage extending deep into the cortex.

Bleaching Your Hair

Lightening your hair a little causes only some damage. Yet radically lightening your hair can damage it severely. An extremely caustic concentration of hydrogen peroxide is needed to go from dark to light in one step. In such concentrations, hydrogen peroxide can burn skin. The peroxide will leave your hair more porous and weak when wet than before it was lightened, so afterward, you can damage your hair simply by running a comb through it. Lightening can also destroy your hair's protein, and there will be little left to hold your hair together after that.

Perming Your Curls

Every time your hair is permed, 10 percent of the bonds holding your hair together are lost—and that's just if things went well. If your hair is relaxed, nearly all of the bonds within your hair are converted into weaker bonds (see chapter 9). Avoid anything that involves hydroxides, such as sodium hydroxide or calcium hydroxide, as if it were a hair-eating virus. At best, your hair will be considerably weaker afterward. At worst, you could end up dissolving or partially dissolving your hair. The only thing to do after that is to cut off what is left.

I know it seems like your hair is full of life and energy, but it isn't alive any more than a piece of fabric is. This doesn't mean that your hair has no personality and doesn't feel full of vibrancy. Springiness is built into the structure of each curl, and your hair seems to radiate joy when it's being treated the way it needs to be. But to believe that your hair is *literally* alive is dangerous to the health of your hair. Because hair is actually like a fabric once it has left your scalp: when your hair is damaged, it stays damaged. There is nothing inside the hair shaft that can repair itself as skin does, just as a towel's fibers can't repair themselves. What's done is done. Conditioners can temporarily coat your hair to make it feel nice and smooth, but that's it. People who tell you that their products can "repair" or "heal" your hair are misleading you. Only living things can heal. How can a conditioner repair your hair? By gluing it back together where it's broken? Magically re-creating new fiber to patch up the broken parts while you're using it in the shower? Don't fall for this gimmick; save your money and your hopes. Once damage is done, it's there for the life of your hair until you cut it off or it breaks off. Nothing can heal damaged hair, no matter how expensive the product is—any more than soaking a length of fabric in herbs, exotic oils, proteins, DNA, or vitamins can heal it. Believing that any product out there can repair damage leads people to think that if they damage their hair, it can always be repaired or healed later—if they can only find the right miracle product to do it. This is simply not true, and no matter how much money you spend on a product to repair your hair, it still can't achieve this. That is why it's so important to learn how to prevent damage in the first place.

Geek Out with Teri

Okay, I'm going to go down to the very foundation of your hair, so I should probably warn you: there's a lot of detail about your curls here. I know I'm a total hair geek, but I think our curly hair is fascinating, and it's important to understand how it's put together so that we can make informed decisions on its behalf. The marvel contained within the amazingly complex structure of the cortex determines why and how your hair curls, how it stretches, how hair sets better with water, why hair reverts when wet or if it's humid outside, and why it takes such harsh chemicals to permanently change your hair's nature. If you examine the building blocks of your hair and what keeps it together, you will discover the frailty, as well as the strength, within your curls. Knowing how your hair works also means you'll be able to distinguish advertising misinformation from the truth.

The Fiber of Your Hair

Keratin, a protein, makes up your hair. It's the same protein that nails, claws, beaks, quills, and hooves are made of. One strand of hair is composed of many unimaginably thin coils of protein twisted together to form bundles. The bundles are grouped together into more bundles to form one rope of keratin—which is what one strand of your hair is.

The units that make up your hair's protein are little groups of atoms known as amino acids. Every hair is built amino acid by amino acid, looking like beads on a string. Each amino acid is like a different type of bead placed in a specific sequence on the string, and it reacts to its neighbors a bit differently. One amino acid might be irresistibly attracted to a particular neighbor down the string from it. When attracted, the two amino acids cling to each other. When one amino clings tightly to the amino down the way, it changes the shape of the string when they get together. Amino acids feel this attraction at regular intervals up and down the strand. When they're all bonded to one another, the pattern they create causes the strand to take the shape of a coil.

This coil is an alpha helix, the same shape our DNA takes. Four of these alpha helices are twisted together into a structure called a protofibril (see the figure on page 35). Eleven protofibrils are twisted together to make up one microfibril (or intermediate filament). Hundreds of microfibrils are bundled together and embedded in a protein-cement matrix to form one macrofibril. Bundles of macrofibrils make up the cortex, the main core of the hair. One strand of hair is about ten macrofibrils across. What this means is that one single strand of your hair is composed of

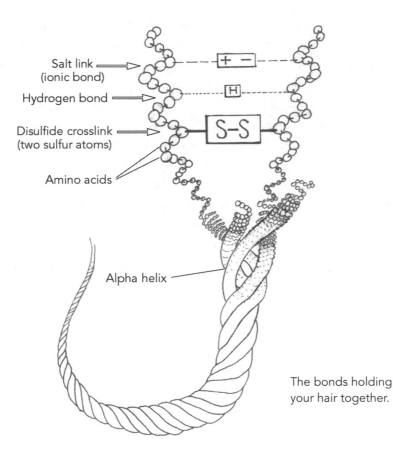

Salt link ⟶
(ionic bond)

Hydrogen bond ⟶

Disulfide crosslink ⟶
(two sulfur atoms)

Amino acids ⟶

Alpha helix ⟶

The bonds holding
your hair together.

hundreds of thousands of surpassingly thin strands of fiber, twisted and bonded together. Every strand of hair you produce is an intricate marvel of construction. (See the illustration on page 29.)

A string of amino acids builds each hair into the twists of an alpha helix. The alpha helix is the building unit of every strand of hair. Because of its coiled nature, when you stretch a strand of hair, the helices unwind to accommodate the stretching without breaking. The strand can unwind to about 30 percent of its length and still return to its previously coiled shape without damage. When stretched, the twisted shape of the helix changes from coils to pleated sheets, like an accordion fold. When released, they spiral back up again.

When your hair is stretched beyond this amount, the helices are stretched too far and break. Knowing this is crucial when you're combing or brushing your hair. When you pull a comb or brush through your hair, your hair is stretched. If you do it gently, it springs right back. If you use lots of force to get a brush or a comb through your hair, such as when your hair isn't slippery enough, the comb's teeth are too close together, or heavy force is exerted to get the comb or the brush through your hair in a hurry, your hair is stretched and damaged. If you use a brush such as a Denman (see chapter 8), which has some give to it because of its flexible rubber base, the give comes from the brush instead of your hair. If you use, or someone uses on you, a hard plastic comb or moves through your hair with force, this means all the give must come from your hair alone. This will damage your hair. Keeping this in mind is a vital way to prevent needless damage getting inflicted on your hair.

The Bonds

Not only do the bonds of each strand of your hair hold it together, but the way these bonds are composed also explains why your hair behaves as it does. The bonds determine how much your hair curls, why it frizzes in humidity, and why a set holds better when it's done with wet hair. There are three main bonds within and between all of those alpha helices that determine the structure and behavior of your hair: hydrogen bonds, salt bonds, and disulfide bonds (see the illustration on page 35). The coils are shaped by the interactions between the bonds, both within their structures and with neighboring coils. These bonds repeat down their entire lengths. Because of their massive numbers, they are powerful.

Why Your Hair Acts Differently When Wet

When your hair gets wet, your tighter curls might seem to relax and your hair seems longer. Hair that is set when wet takes and holds its set much better than the same hair that is set when dry. Your hair is also more vulnerable at this time. What does water do to your hair to make it change, and why is it that water can undo the very style that it helped set?

Wet Hair

I used to find it so frustrating when I was younger and wore my hair texturized. I believed it looked so much better when it was wet because my curls were defined then. It looked longer, it hung with a nice weight, it swung around when I moved my head, and the curls seemed like they were taking it easy instead of being their usual clenched selves (at that time I wished for looser curls). I spent many years trying to figure out a way to get my hair to act like it was wet when it was dry. Perhaps this was the big appeal of the unfortunate Jheri curl. All that oil made hair seem permanently wet—which in a way it was, but with oil. I've since discovered that using a conditioner as described later in this book actually makes dry hair act more like it does when it's wet. The great part about it is that your hair will look dry, but, unlike with the Jheri curl, it's touchable.

When your hair gets wet, water molecules break the hydrogen bonds in your hair by inserting themselves between the bonds. With water inserted between the hydrogen bonds, hair loosens and extends. Your hair is weaker when wet because the hydrogen bonds that reinforced it have been broken. With less reinforcement in the hair fiber, your hair needs to be handled even more carefully when wet. Your hair can absorb 30 percent of its weight in water, so it's now heavier as well. With the additional water weight added to it and with the hydrogen bonds temporarily broken, curly wet hair hangs longer and has looser curls than when dry.

When you wet-set your hair, your hair is held in this extended position while it dries and the hydrogen bonds return. The hydrogen bonds re-form with your hair in the new, stretched-out position. The re-formed hydrogen atoms will hold in their new extended positions until water is introduced again, either in the shower, in the rain, or in high humidity. The hydrogen atoms will then break apart again, and when they break apart, they'll settle back either to their default positions of your natural curl pattern (determined by the disulfide bonds) or into the positions determined by a new set. In this way, hydrogen atoms behave much like a swarm of flies. They can be shooed away by water but will return and land on whatever attractive surfaces they can find.

Even small amounts of water can create a big change in the appearance of your hair. Humid air can make your curls lose definition and expand as if they were filled with helium. How does humid air tighten up your curls without a drop of water touching them?

Humidity and You

Humidity brings out the cloudlike qualities of our hair. Although humidity affects many people's hair enough to give them "fly-aways" or make their ends fluffier, humidity can make our hair expand to the point that it might take up an entire doorway. Our curls seem to explode apart, in slow motion, enough to startle passersby. Many times we may want to play up our hair's spectacular expansive nature (and I have several styles showcasing this in chapter 13), but at other times you may want to simply get through the day with predictable hair. If this is the case, it's good to understand what humidity does with your hair.

Angela Nissel vividly described her hair's reaction to humidity. She wrote in *Mixed: My Life in Black and White*, "My hair expands like a balloon if there is any humidity. If the kid sitting next to me spills his juice box—poof—the liquid on the floor causes my hair to enlarge. Every single day I'd leave the house with two braids and two barrettes, and sometime between the Pledge of Allegiance and the first bathroom break one of my barrettes would pop off, unable to sustain my swelling, expanding hair."

You might be able to shield your hair from rain, but humidity is present everywhere that air is present. When it's extremely humid, there is a high percentage of water in the air, which means there is a reservoir of hydrogen available. If your hair has been flattened or set while wet, hydrogen atoms were removed and re-formed in new positions as the hair dried. When hydrogen atoms are absorbed back into your hair from the humidity, they return to all of the old positions they'd been removed from when your hair was set. As the hydrogen atoms return, they reinforce and tighten each twist and curl. As strands of hair take in hydrogen, the curls draw up at slightly different rates or in varying amounts. Sometimes hair that's closer to the outside is exposed to the humidity before hair near your scalp is. As the hairs spread apart, your curls no longer lie perfectly in sync with one another. Now, with each strand's natural curl returning, it's happily doing its own thing. With each strand behaving independently, your entire head of hair blows up.

If all of this sounds hauntingly familiar, don't worry. This book will teach you how to prevent your hair from expanding in humid weather if you don't want it to. (See chapter 6.)

What Makes Your Hair Curl Like It Does?

I do beadwork. Some of the projects I've done needed some sort of filling to form a three-dimensional shape before I would bead over it. I don't trust synthetic batting, so I use my own hair. I get the hair from my comb to stuff smaller projects. It's natural, I know where it comes from, and no synthetic battings are hurt in the making of my project. It's also like stamping a project as truly mine to put my own hair in it. Plus, my hair is so spongy that it makes the *perfect* batting material. I'd save for a month or two to get enough hair to stuff my project properly.

Once I was making a purse with raised faces that I was stuffing with my hair, and right as I was about to finish, I ran low on hair. My friend Brewster had just had his hair cut, and he offered me a handful of his straight blond hair. It was free hair, so I reasoned, What the heck.

When I use my own hair, I ball it up and simply stuff it into a little opening in my project with a chopstick, and it stays. Brewster's hair was totally different. First, I had to fold it in half, and it *did not* want to fold. It also didn't want to go into the hole in my project. Once I'd wrangled it into the opening by force and determination, it kept trying to pop out. It was a challenge to sew the project shut with all that blond hair trying to slip out. Even after the bag was sewn shut and beaded over, more than a decade later, I still see little flaxen hairs determinedly working their way out of the bag.

My experience with our two opposite hair types demonstrated how different our hair was. They acted like two entirely different substances. I have since found out that they are indeed built differently, right down to the types of cells they have.

The Shape of Your Follicles

There are several factors that make your hair so curly: curls are shaped by the follicles they grow from, by the uneven rate each side of the hair grows, and by the composition of the cells within each twist and turn of the curl. Curls are built deep into every fiber of hair and are structurally reinforced by the placement of the cells within them.

The shape of your follicles determines how much your hair curls, much as a squirt of cake frosting is changed by the shape of the tip it's squeezed from. Straight hair comes from a rounded follicle and is nearly round in cross section. Wavy hair comes from a slightly oval follicle, so the hair that grows from it is slightly oval. Loosely curled hair comes from a more oval follicle, and in cross section looks oval. Very curly hair, such as is common in those of us of African descent, has follicles that are like flattened ovals. In cross section, each of our hairs is bean-shaped to nearly flat, and grows from its follicle like a ribbon. Very curly African American hair can have up to thirty more twists per inch than Caucasian hair has.

Uneven Growth

It's believed that our hair may curl the way it does because one side of it grows faster than the other side. This uneven rate of growth would cause it to somersault determinedly over itself. If one side is longer than the other, hair will always be more comfortable in a curled position, rather than pulled straight.

I had no idea about this until I started to do some deep digging while I researched hair. Two basic types of cells make up the cortex. The really

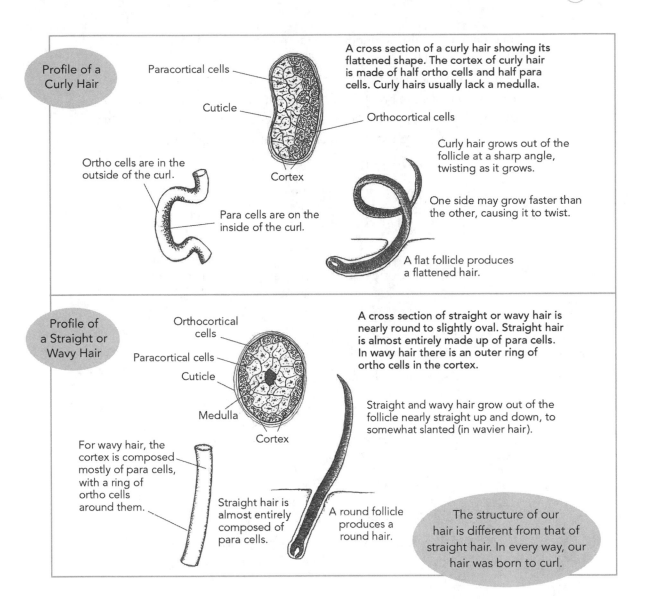

Profile of a Curly Hair

Paracortical cells

Cuticle

Orthocortical cells

Cortex

A cross section of a curly hair showing its flattened shape. The cortex of curly hair is made of half ortho cells and half para cells. Curly hairs usually lack a medulla.

Ortho cells are in the outside of the curl.

Para cells are on the inside of the curl.

Curly hair grows out of the follicle at a sharp angle, twisting as it grows.

One side may grow faster than the other, causing it to twist.

A flat follicle produces a flattened hair.

Profile of a Straight or Wavy Hair

Orthocortical cells

Paracortical cells

Cuticle

Medulla

Cortex

A cross section of straight or wavy hair is nearly round to slightly oval. Straight hair is almost entirely made up of para cells. In wavy hair there is an outer ring of ortho cells in the cortex.

Straight and wavy hair grow out of the follicle nearly straight up and down, to somewhat slanted (in wavier hair).

For wavy hair, the cortex is composed mostly of para cells, with a ring of ortho cells around them.

Straight hair is almost entirely composed of para cells.

A round follicle produces a round hair.

The structure of our hair is different from that of straight hair. In every way, our hair was born to curl.

interesting thing is that in curly hair, they are present in different amounts and are placed differently from the way they are in people who have straight or wavy hair. These two types of cells are called the orthocortical cells and the paracortical cells. Straight hair is almost entirely composed of paracortical cells. Wavy hair is mostly paracortical cells, with a thin ring of orthocortical cells surrounding them. Very curly hair is made up of half orthocortical and half paracortical cells.

Our bodies put an unimaginable amount of work into creating each and every spiraled hair we grow. Every coil on our heads is made from infinitesimally tiny fibers, packed thousands of times over into every strand. Our curls are deeply curled, and they are built, atom upon atom, to curl the

TAKE AWAY Tips

- Hair is like a delicate fabric. The more gently you treat it, the longer it lasts.

- Your hair was made to curl. Curls are built into every twist of your hair by the shape of your follicles, the rate that each side grows, and the types of cells within your hair.

- Treat your hair as you do your skin. If it hurts your skin, it hurts your hair.

- The thinner your individual strands of hair, the more gently you must treat them.

- Hair will grow to its maximum length if it isn't being damaged. On average, this means it will reach at least to your lower back.

- Hair that is stretched too far, such as when you're combing or brushing it roughly or using an unforgiving comb, will break.

- If a product can't heal or repair a sweater that's soaked in it, it won't repair or heal your hair either.

- Multiply whatever you're doing to your hair by the hundreds (or thousands) of times it will happen over the lifetime of your hair to determine its true effect on your hair.

- Hair doesn't grow because we find a quick gimmick to make it grow. It grows after we learn how to take care of it and stop hurting it.

way they do. Our curls are a genetic bridge to the curls of those who have come before us, embedded deep in our DNA to coil as they do.

So, now you've seen how your curly hair is built, inside and out, and why its shape and thickness make it behave as it does. You've also learned where and how damage occurs on your hair and its effect. Now that you know how your hair is put together, it's time to learn the seven steps to take care of it in a way that doesn't damage it anymore: shampoo, condition, comb, define, dry, protect, and refresh.

Chapter Three

Shampooing
Washing without the Matting

When my mom was away at college, washing her hair was such a daunting process that she would wait for school breaks to come home and have her mom do it for her. The hair-care rules that work for people with straight hair often don't apply to those of us with very curly hair. Our hair behaves differently from hair that has only waves and slight curls. Tight curls are creatures unto themselves, and because of this, our curls need to be shampooed differently from the way other hair types do. We must shampoo our hair in a way that takes account of our tight ringlets. To do otherwise wastes many hours of effort as we try to turn a mat back into hair.

I've found several strategies that will help your curls stay healthy and vibrant, while still letting them be their quirky selves. These techniques allow you to showcase your curls in the most flattering way, emphasizing their uniqueness. What I've found is that keeping your hair as calm as possible goes a long way in working *with* your curly nature.

Your curls are easily excited and flustered. How you treat your curls when washing them sets the tone for how they will react to you when you comb them out. In this chapter, I'll share several techniques you can try at each stage of washing and rinsing to keep your coils as soothed and contented as possible. Learning how to shampoo your curls properly is the first step to their health.

You Don't Need to Shampoo Every Day

Curls are delicate, and they want only to be treated with patience and kindness. Most of all, they need to be handled with an understanding of their unique nature. Unless you have a very oily scalp, you don't need to shampoo every time you take a shower. And, in fact, there are many who don't use shampoo at all, but use a conditioner in its place (for more about this option, see chapter 7). Shampooing every day will dry out and wear out your curls. This is especially true if you consider that every shampoo will most likely mean a combing as well. Working your hair so often is damaging. It's best to handle curly hair as infrequently as possible in order to grow it long.

Always keep in mind that shampooing is for your scalp only. People with straighter hair tend to wash their hair every day because their hair gets oily by the next day and looks flat. We don't have that issue. Because our hair is very curly and tends to be extremely dry, it doesn't get oily from our scalps. Only if you put lots of oily products on your hair might it need washing more often. I've found the best results to be washing and combing my hair every four to seven days. After seven days, the curls tend to get more tangled, and it takes more time to comb them. Combing them sooner than every four days keeps them in a constant tizzy; my curls are just getting settled in from their last combing when they're put through the whole process again if I comb more often than every four days. Not to mention all of the additional, unnecessary wear and tear.

Save Time by Combing Less

The more often you comb, the less time you actually spend combing at each session, but the process doesn't become time effective at a certain frequency of combing. Here's my logic: I've found that it takes about thirty minutes to recomb freshly combed hair. This means that if I comb my hair all the way through, set the comb down for a few seconds, then pick it back up and start combing once again, it will take me about thirty minutes the second time. So, no matter how often I comb my hair, it will take a minimum of half an hour each time. I've found that when I comb my hair every four days, it takes about an hour to comb. If I go seven days, it takes about two hours to comb.

This means that if I spend at least thirty minutes combing my hair every day, at the end of the week, I will have spent a minimum of three and a half hours combing that week. Not to mention the time it takes to wash, rinse, and condition my hair, then the four-plus hours to air-dry it. (I highly discourage blow-drying it every day because of the rapidly mounting damage this causes.) Most of my week would then be spent on my hair. So this doesn't seem like the most practical option.

By this same reasoning, combing every four days would seem to be ideal. Combing every four days takes me a little more than an hour each time, so I would spend a bit less than two hours a week combing it (two hours every eight days). Shampooing and combing about twice a week keeps my curls nice and fresh looking. The downside, I've found, is that I would spend more time washing and drying it—I'd have to do this about twice a week—but it's challenging to stay on schedule. Every four days means it would be a different weekday to wash my hair, and washing during the week is inconvenient. I always manage to forget or put it off until the next day, then the next day, and the next, and before I know it, more than a week and a half has passed, and then I have a mess to get through.

So shampooing and combing every seven days has worked out for me. I have one set day each week when I wash and comb my hair, and I can plan for it. I can stay in and watch TV or a movie while I comb, then run errands while it dries.

The Strategy: Keeping Your Hair as Calm as Possible while Shampooing

When you handle your coiled hair, the most important rule is to keep it as smooth and calm as possible, at all times, always. Your curls are high-strung and need to be treated as gently as possible. This especially goes for washing, when your spirals are wet and vulnerable.

On television or in movies, actors are often shown in the shower gathering their hair onto the top of their heads and lathering it vigorously into a foamy mass. Straight hair by its nature lies flat. So, even after being scrunched into a soapy ball and rubbed into a lather fit for laundry, it takes only a bit of combing to make it flat and straight again. It might be tempting to wash your hair the way you see it being done on TV or in the movies. Although it does look glamorous on screen, the result for you would be the opposite of glamour. You would be left with a compressed hair-lump attached to your head where curls once lived.

Know that shampoo commercials and shower scenes in movies are almost exclusively meant for people with straighter hair, even when they happen to be showing a model of color and/or with curly hair. I have found that the media are very straight-hair blinded, as if tightly curly hair doesn't exist. The only time I've seen tightly curled hair talked about in the media is in commercials that push relaxers or flat irons—which doesn't make me feel better. At all. Maybe it's a matter of convenience. Maybe it's easier than writing into the script how the protagonist washes her hair in a way that's certain to tangle it, then must sit down to comb it for several hours, as a consequence of washing it that way, before the action can continue. The media's portrayal of hair affects how we view our own hair. It's human nature to compare. Since childhood, we've been gauging ourselves against others, even if we don't want to. When we watch television and see that there are *no* representations of hair that behaves like ours, it's easy for us to feel as if we aren't normal. To inoculate ourselves against these stealthy influences, we need to be aware of this media bias toward straight hair. If you are, it will save you the energy you would otherwise waste by feeling bad about your hair. Especially since you have magnificent, unique hair—and that's a good thing. As soon as you know how to emphasize your spirals, people will be coming up to you to admire them. They'll tell you they haven't seen anything like your hair.

During the few times that curly hair is mentioned in the media, even when it's referred to as "extremely curly," they still mean mildly curly hair at best. We are repeatedly shown that the only way to handle *all* hair is by using the methods that work with straighter hair. When I was growing up, I felt as if there were only two options for all hair types: either you lucked out and the methods worked for you, or you were unlucky and they didn't.

I recently saw a television show featuring a beautiful actress of mixed ethnicity who has hair that's nearly as curly as mine. In the show, she swam with her hair down. Then she got out of the water, towel dried, and got dressed, swinging her hair around— and just like that, it looked perfectly combed, and she was out the door. Now, if I'd seen this when I was a kid while trying to figure out my own hair, I would have felt a pain in my heart. I would have strongly identified with this actress and her beautiful hair. Then to see her treat her hair exactly as people with straighter hair do, I would have felt even more aberrant. I would have been convinced that something really was wrong with me because my hair took an hour-plus at that time to comb.

So I need to tell you this: First, your tightly curled hair is totally normal, and it's beautiful. Second, I've recently seen several crafting programs that showed how to make felt out of wool. The wool fibers are placed touching one another or knitted together, then they're dunked in soapy water. Once they're saturated, the fibers are rubbed until they lock together into felt. Once the fibers have been felted, they are permanently locked together. And this got me thinking that if you pile up your hair and rub shampoo into it, you're basically felting your hair. Felt is great for a hat but not so flattering as hair. This means that if you have curly hair, *never, ever* pile it on top of your head and rub it into a sudsy pile. At best, you will have a mess. Most likely, you'll end up with a matted mass, and it could take hours to even locate the ends of your hair to begin to comb it out. Curly hair must be treated differently from straight hair. (I know I keep saying it, but this idea is crucial. Plus, I have to counteract all the years of media brainwashing that most of us have probably endured about how to handle our hair.)

There are two different styling goals for straight hair and for very curly hair, and they are opposed to each other. Straight hair is flat and tends to become limp. It's easily weighed down. All products and hair-care techniques that are meant for this type of hair are designed to help give it a bit more life and volume.

Curly hair is buoyant by its nature and has an abundance of volume. It naturally expands and fluffs up. The goal with curly hair is to calm it down, soothe it, and emphasize its lovely texture. *Curly hair must be treated like curly hair.* The goal when washing your curly hair is to keep it as smooth and calm as possible. Tangling is in the nature of our curls. Give them no additional reasons to tangle. Your hair will thank you.

Shampooing Overview: Focus on Your Scalp

The best way to shampoo your hair is to apply shampoo only to your scalp. This is because curly hair is very dry. The sebum from your scalp almost never makes its way down the twists in your curls. Even if it does, it doesn't make a bit of difference; curly hair has volume to spare. Your curls won't notice that tiny bit of weight. Tight curls can handle oils being left on them, because a little weight is a good thing.

Shampoo is meant to clean your scalp because it's your scalp that produces the oil. Your hair will still get clean from the shampoo that is applied to your scalp. The sudsy water will run down your hair as it's rinsed off. Directly shampooing the ends of your curly hair is harsh and drying— and unnecessary. Following are some recommended ways to cleanse all of your hair, but, happily, these techniques will keep your ends moist and conditioned.

How to Shampoo Those Curls while Keeping Them Calm

The first step in shampooing is to let the water run over your hair for a minute or two. Keep your hair hanging down and as smooth as possible. This saturates your hair, ensures that it's soaked, yet keeps your ends smooth. Because curly hair is thick, you might need to give the water time to soak in. To help it along, gently place your fingers under your hair to lift it off your scalp. This gives the water a leg up, figuratively speaking, to reach all the way through your hair. Also, poke your fingers through your hair and open it up in places to make sure the water gets all the way in.

Once your hair has been saturated, take a small palmful of mild shampoo or a cleansing conditioner (see chapter 11 for recommended products) and rub your hands together, making sure your fingers are coated. Smooth the shampoo onto your scalp only, by inserting your fingers *beneath* your hair. This way, your hair has as little direct contact with the shampoo as possible.

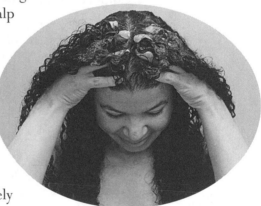

Now gently rub the shampoo into your scalp, *under* your hair, so that you don't disturb your hair. Remember, shampooing is for your scalp. It's your scalp that gets oily. Your hair is an innocent bystander. Use only the balls of your fingers, never your nails, which will merely scrape your scalp.

Rub your scalp from beneath your hair. This keeps your hair from getting matted.

When your scalp has been lathered, it's time to rinse. It's important to rinse your hair thoroughly. Help the water get into your hair so that it can do its job. Slide your fingers under your hair at your hairline, and lift your hair up a little. Let the water flow through your hair while you make small, cautious openings to ensure that it's flushed with water. Your ends should be hanging straight down during every step. Your curly hair can be quite thick, and without conditioner it behaves as a solid mass does. Be especially gentle at this time.

While your hair is being rinsed, watered-down shampoo will flow through it. This, along with the next step, will clean your hair thoroughly, but the next step will moisturize it at the same time.

The After Rinse: Shampoo, Rinse, Repeat—Improved

The after-rinse step ensures that your ends are fresh and clean, but—surprisingly—moisturized, too. This step uses a conditioner instead of the misguided second shampooing that is often recommended on most bottles of shampoo. Your conditioner will step in to perform the role that's usually played by the shampoo. By swapping conditioner for shampoo, you're still using something that will grab and hold onto any remaining dirt or excess oils. Conditioner can attach itself to grime as well as shampoo does. The conditioner will take the grime down the drain with it as you rinse it off. The big advantage here is that you've bypassed the harsh drying that comes from a second shampooing and replaced it with something healthy.

I do this last cleansing of my hair before the final application of real conditioner. It ensures that my scalp is clean and my hair well rinsed. This is especially helpful if my hair happens to be very dirty. If it is, I add more rinsing conditioner and really poke and squeeze it all through my hair. The advantage is that if I have to do it several times for some reason (sprayed by a skunk, sand poured into my hair), it's no big thing. Because I am using conditioner, I can repeat as many times as necessary.

Rinsing with conditioner is an optional step, but it's a healthy substitute if shampoo is trapped inside the matted areas and it's hard to get it out of there. Like a mole, the conditioner likes to burrow in tangled spots. This conditioning rinse lubricates your hair and helps loosen your mats so that it's easier to rinse your hair.

What about a Pre-Poo?

A pre-poo is when you cover the ends of your hair with conditioner, to protect them, before you shampoo your hair. This is a fine practice; however, it isn't necessary when you use the techniques I've described, because with a step that comes later on your ends will already be covered in conditioner. So adding more conditioner on top of the conditioner that's already in your hair would be redundant, plus a waste of conditioner.

Note: If your hair is difficult to handle all at once, you can pin up one half and do the other half first, then take it down and do the second half. This is what I do.

Use a small palmful of conditioner (see "The Real Portions for Curls" on page 59) and rub it into your scalp under your hair, as if it were shampoo. You need to use a generous amount—your curls are thick, and more is needed to coat them. Squeeze more conditioner into the ends of your hair. Once your hair is coated, knead it by squeezing up and down your hair. When you see the conditioner "sploot" between your fingers, you'll know you've used enough.

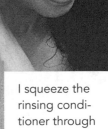

I squeeze the rinsing conditioner through each half of my hair.

When your hair has been coated, rinse out the conditioner. Gently work your hair open in little patches, as you did with the shampoo. Never pull your hair apart all the way to the ends, like a wishbone. Open it in little spots to let the water flow in, then move on to other areas. The conditioner makes your hair slippery, so any shampoo that's trapped inside a thick tangled spot can be reached with ease. Now you are ready for the next step: conditioning.

I make sure the rinsing conditioner is rinsed out by making small openings in my hair for the water to flow through.

Money-Saving Tips for Using Extra Shampoo and Conditioners

You've probably bought a few shampoos and conditioners that didn't work for your hair. If you're like me, you might feel a little guilty throwing out most of the bottle just because you can't use it on your head. Here are some tricks I've learned over the years to use up those bottles of product I can't seem to get myself to throw out.

Cleaning Makeup Brushes

I learned this tip from a person behind a department store makeup counter: you can use these shampoos to clean makeup brushes. Rinse your makeup brush in warm water, apply a little dab of shampoo to the brush, and rub it gently into a lather. Rinse and dry your brush. The first person to look over my book shared another great idea: put shampoo that doesn't work so well on your hair into a hand-soap pump bottle to wash your hands with.

Rinsing Conditioners That Didn't Work?

I use conditioners that would have sat on my shelf unused or even been tossed out as my rinsing conditioners. Perhaps some of these conditioners didn't contain enough emollients for my combing or I didn't like their scents or I'd bought them because I loved their scent, but they turned out to be too watery for setting my curls. If you're using a cleansing conditioner (conditioners sold specifically to use in place of shampoos), you could try a cleansing conditioner that's meant more for your scalp during the shampooing step, and use another one that's more emollient-based for the after-rinse step.

Deep Scrub

You can use these same lighter conditioners for a deep body scrub. I have to say that I'm a cleanser-and-water kind of person. I haven't seen any benefit in using fancy products, so I try to use what I have creatively. I use a washcloth or one of those poofy nylon puffs and a light conditioner (or conditioner mixed with body wash to make it more mild) to scrub over my body once or twice a week. Because the conditioner is slippery, I don't get washcloth burn. I also don't dry out my skin. When I rinse off the conditioner after scrubbing with the washcloth, my skin feels smooth and somewhat moisturized but not too much. You could also try this using baking soda as your scrub.

I know that you are aware of this, but I do want to add that as with any product, you should avoid your eye area, and if you're sensitive to scents, some ingredients, or certain preservatives, please check the labels before trying this scrub.

Shaving

You can also use conditioner as a shaving cream. If you ever find yourself on a trip and you don't have (or didn't have room to pack) shaving cream, use your conditioner in its place. Slather the conditioner on as you would shaving cream, and then shave it off. I love conditioner. If I were on a desert island, conditioner would be the one household item I'd choose to bring with me.

Cleansing Can Be Moisturizing After All

If you know how to shampoo your hair without matting it, and you use conditioner to clean your hair while keeping it moisturized, then shampooing will be a healthy treatment for your hair, instead of a process that dries it out. Shampooing and using a conditioner as a rinse make the shampooing process one less opportunity to damage your hair. The second step in the seven steps to happy hair, conditioning, primes your curls to be the striking spirals they were born to be.

TAKE AWAY Tips

- Always keep your hair smooth when cleansing.
- Wet your hair thoroughly by letting water run over it.
- Shampoo is for your scalp. Apply shampoo only to your scalp.
- Lather *under* your hair.
- Use only the pads of your fingers.
- Rinse, and then apply a light conditioner to cleanse without stripping your hair. Smooth it over your scalp and hair, then rinse again.

Chapter Four

Conditioning
How to Get Unflappable Curls

When I was about fifteen, I thought I'd finally found the perfect shampoo and conditioner. The shampoo was thick and smelled faintly of oranges and seemed not to dry my hair as much as other shampoos did. The conditioner was the consistency of mayonnaise, and I thought that any month now, I'd be able to see my hair actually make it past the shoulder barrier. To be sure this happened, I bought a little jar of the deep conditioner in the product line and used it, too. Although my hair didn't grow, one day as I prepared my hair for school, I noticed that it was sticky. It felt like a mist of rubber cement had been sprayed over it. So, it wasn't only crunchy now, but sticky. On that morning, it had progressed to gummy. Being a teenage girl, I was mortified. What on earth was my hair doing to me now? How could I go to school with hair that felt like a sticky note?

I was in a bad mood all day and snapped at everyone. I kept touching my hair and growing more upset. My homework papers and the pages of my schoolbooks began to stick to my fingers. Finally, a kind teacher pulled me aside and asked what was going on. I told her about the mind game I suspected my hair was playing on me. She asked whether I'd been using the same shampoo and conditioner every time I washed my hair. When I said yes, she said it was most likely product buildup. I was relieved that this wasn't a new torture my hair had thought up for me. Yet it meant that my beloved products couldn't be relied on every time I washed. So I was back to the drawing board, looking for the magic products to "cure" my hair. (It turns out those products contained the "sticky" ingredients I learned from this incident to avoid. I'll talk more about ingredients to avoid in chapter 11.)

Of course, I never found those magic products. There are none. Damage done can't be undone, no matter what sweet promises a bottle might whisper seductively to you. Ten years later my hair grew long, but only after I stopped hurting it with caustic perms. This isn't to say that having a good product and knowing how best to use it can't work wonders. It turns out that the "wonder product" I'd been searching for had been with me the whole time, much like Dorothy's shoes in *The Wizard of Oz*. It's a regular bottle of conditioner, available from any drugstore. I simply had to stop destroying my hair and then learn a new way to use that conditioner.

Putting in conditioner preps your hair for combing, one of the most crucial steps toward having manageable, conditioned spirals. This is the third step that readies your hair to form into perfectly separated curls. It also fortifies your hair to withstand wind, humidity, and being slept on and styled in the morning. After vigorous activity, your hair won't explode into a mushroom cloud (unless you *choose* for it to be a cloud—by gently finger-combing it apart—to show off its texture). Using conditioner the way I describe in this chapter will highlight every unique twist in every curl, uniting all of your strands in place. Although very much in control, your curls won't be crunchy, as they would be with gel or mousse. They'll simply feel like they grew that way.

The Real Portions for Curls

The miserly portions recommended by nearly every hair-care product I've ever used have often misled me. The suggested portions seem to be meant for people with doll-size heads. The truth for us curly girls is that those tiny sizes aren't meant for our hair, but for limp hair that collapses with the slightest amount of weight. Our hair is different, so an entirely different set of rules applies. The suggested portions would be but a helpless drop in the sea of our hair. When reading the suggested amount of conditioner on the bottle (for laughs), I usually think, There, there, isn't that adorable? What a precious amount! Look how cute. They think my hair would even notice a dime-size portion like that.

Then I squeeze out a copious, healthy amount of conditioner into my palm—the size of which has nothing whatsoever to do with their recommended portion. Remember, those directions were not written for your curls. They were written for wimpy, lifeless hair that's easily deflated, *not* for your vigorous, spirited coils that laugh in the face of a little conditioner. *You* have to use enough for your hair to notice.

This is very important: If you think you put in too much conditioner, then that should be just about the right amount. It's best to use roughly a palmful of conditioner for each half of your hair, especially if it's longer than shoulder-length as well as thick (or very long or extremely thick). This might sound like a huge amount at first, but your thick curls *need* lots of conditioner. They also absorb much more conditioner than flat or wavy hair does. It's better to err on the side of too much conditioner, because it self-regulates. Try to use too much, and see what happens. If you put on too much, it'll be combed out while you're combing your hair. When I put in conditioner, it glops all over everything. By the time I'm done combing, the conditioner has disappeared; it's been combed into my hair.

Be bold and experiment. Know that if you put too little in, your curls won't have the weight and control they need. And you probably won't discover this until your hair is dry, and you're noticing that it looks a bit fuzzy and your curls are beginning to puff apart. It can be fixed at that point, but not easily.

The main point is, you won't know all the wonders that conditioner can do for your hair unless you have enough of it in there. True, until you get used to using the healthy portions that are meant for thick curls, it might *seem* like too much. Remember, though, most of the conditioner is water, so the bulk of it will evaporate. That's why you need to apply plenty of it. This way, once your hair has dried, ample portions of the other ingredients are left behind to do their magic. You'll find that you can use much more conditioner than you realized. The trick is to use a lot. Too little, and it won't make much of a difference in your thick curls.

In addition to weighing down longer curls and giving them touchable control, the conditioner also moisturizes your hair. You'll no longer need hairdressing if you used it before. Suddenly, with the proper use of conditioner, your hair will be touchable and moisturized but not greasy. I found that using conditioner in this way truly revolutionized how my hair behaved. It was the final piece of the puzzle.

I talk about the best conditioners in chapter 11, but if you are impatient like me, you probably want to know of a few now. The conditioners I recommend are the ones that work with these techniques. There are many conditioners with ingredients that build up, get crunchy or sticky, or are too watery, but these are just right:

- Aussie Moist
- Clairol Herbal Essences Hello Hydration, None of Your Frizzness, Totally Twisted, or Break's Over conditioners
- Paula's Choice Daily Conditioner (available at CosmeticsCop.com)
- Shikai's Natural Everyday Conditioner

For a longer list of the best conditioners to use, see chapter 11 or TightlyCurly.com.

Applying Conditioner

When the after-shampoo conditioner has been rinsed out of your hair, it's time to put in the real conditioner. To ensure that you can evenly distribute the conditioner, divide long or very thick hair loosely in half, without forcing it, and work on each half separately. (If your hair is very thick or very tangled, it might need to be gently divided into three or four more manageable sections. This makes it easier to distribute the conditioner.)

Here are some tips for using your conditioner in a whole new way. Take a *healthy* palmful of conditioner and glop it onto the first half of your hair. Start about an inch or two from your scalp and work it completely into your hair, all the while keeping your hair hanging down and smooth. Move your fingers in and out of the most tangled spots and smooth the conditioner to the ends. Treat each half like one unified object, as if you were conditioning a wet sweater, rather than trying to run your fingers through your hair.

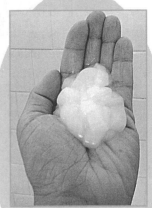

I use one full palmful of conditioner for half of my hair.

It's best to start smoothing on the conditioner about an inch or two from your scalp. This is because your scalp produces its own oils, which will easily travel that inch or so of new hair (provided that your hair isn't damaged by chemicals). Usually, your hair here is the strongest. Because it's recently emerged, newly made from your scalp, it's been exposed to few stresses that would cause damage. In addition, conditioner will be worked up to your scalp as you comb through the hair near your scalp after combing the ends. Your scalp is the one place that can get overwhelmed with too much product (and the follicles may even get damaged with too much product buildup), and since it doesn't really need it anyway, it's best to start a couple inches down on your hair.

The big exception to this is if you've recently started to grow out a perm, and the two hair textures meet near your scalp. In that case, work the conditioner well, but gently, into the tangled spots. Poke your conditioner-laden fingers through your hair to evenly distribute the conditioner, and make sure the more matted sections that need lubricating get it.

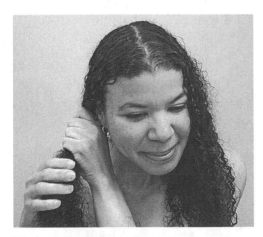

Working the final conditioner in.

Once the conditioner has been worked through to your hair's ends, gently squeeze it into your hair. Knead it like a bag full of frosting. Squeezing helps push the conditioner into the tangled spots. Poke your fingers into areas that feel matted. Make sure you feel the conditioner sploot out from between your fingers when you squeeze, so that you know your hair is saturated.

When your curls are slathered with conditioner, twist that half of your hair into a loose bun if it's long, or if your hair is shorter, clip it up to keep it out of your way. Don't make the buns too tight, because this will squeeze out all of your conditioner, and you need every bit to do its job properly.

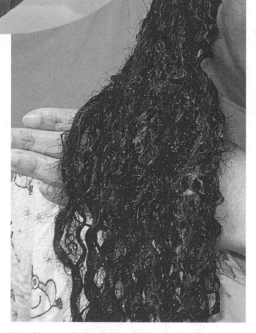

The second handful of conditioner I put in the other half of my hair. I've found that it's difficult to use too much.

After you finish conditioning the first half of your hair, apply another *full* palmful to the second half of your hair. Then squeeze it through the second side, again poking conditioner into the matted parts.

When both halves of your hair have been thoroughly filled with conditioner and pinned or twisted out of the way, you can finish your shower. This way, any conditioner that falls on you can be washed off, and your hair is out of the way.

It's best if you don't towel-dry your hair. You need your hair soaking wet for two reasons: to get the comb through it and for the conditioner to do its work. When I comb, I put on a comfy pajama top to soak up any water and conditioner. By the time I'm finished with the process, my hair is just damp.

My hair is thoroughly saturated with water and conditioner.

This is important: Do not rinse the conditioner out of your hair. The conditioner has much work ahead of it, keeping your curls conditioned and, if you like defined curls as I do, frizz free. Yet it can work only if it's in your hair and not flowing down the drain.

The Magic of Leaving the Conditioner In

Leaving conditioner in your hair coats each strand with emollients and smoothing ingredients. By leaving conditioner in your hair, you no longer need hairdressings, frizz serums, or lotions. Leaving conditioner in will transform your curls into smooth-and-defined-nongreasy-able-to-withstand-humidity-wind-rain-and-moves-when-you-move-your-head curls. Also, when whole curls are clumped together, the *individual* hairs within those curls are shielded from damage. Instead of each lone strand being exposed to the elements, the strands will all act as a unit, where no one strand is exposed. Many strands will be completely encased in hairs, like a cocoon, therefore totally protected. This means that at any one time, the majority of your hair strands are shielded from the elements.

Remember, growing longer, manageable hair is like knowing the combination to a lock. These techniques work together to give you healthy hair that's weatherproof and predictable. But the lock won't open if you use only some of the numbers, or if you don't spin the special number twice. These techniques work only when you use them together. For example, you can use all of the conditioner in the world and buy the exact brands I suggest, but if you rinse it out, or if you don't release and smooth your curls in some way, your hair won't be as manageable, and it sure won't be weatherproof. After cleansing and conditioning, the following chapter covers combing, the step that gives you the perfect canvas to showcase your stunning coils.

Leaving in conditioner will:

- Keep your curls defined
- Help give your curls weight
- Help weatherproof your hair
- Moisturize your hair

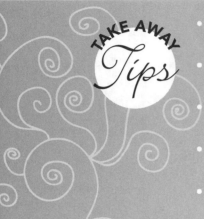

TAKE AWAY Tips

- Keep your hair as smooth and flat as possible when handling it.

- Use a full palmful of conditioner for each half of your hair.

- Apply conditioner by squeezing and poking it into your hair.

- Leave the conditioner in to prime your hair for combing.

- Leave your hair sopping wet for combing. Don't even touch it with a towel.

Chapter Five

Combing

For Those of Us Who Have Ever Gotten a Brush Stuck in Our Hair

Once, when I lived in Santa Cruz, I decided to try a deep-conditioning treatment at a salon. Before I made the appointment, I asked whether they dealt with extremely curly hair. They thought it an odd question but assured me that they did. On meeting the person who would do my hair, I first asked whether he'd worked with extremely curly hair such as mine before. He told me unreservedly that he had. He said he had very personal experience with super-curly hair because he had a friend with hair like mine. Surprised and reassured, I agreed to give the treatment a try. He applied the deep conditioner, spread it in, and had me sit under a hair dryer for half an hour. So far, so good.

When it was time to rinse out the conditioner, the stylist began to scrub at my hair a little vigorously. Feeling paranoid, I again asked whether he had experience combing out really curly hair. I figured that since he'd now actually felt my curls, he'd know whether mine were tighter than the friend's hair he was familiar with. With a laugh, he said he had a trick he used with his friend to comb her hair, and it made combing really easy. Now I was excited. I felt as if I stood before magic gates that were about to open and reveal to me a long-sought treasure—I stood at the threshold of the solution to one of my biggest problems: how to comb my hair easily. And all for the mere price of a deep-conditioning treatment! I would be extra impressed, too, because he was now rubbing my hair enthusiastically, which isn't something a person familiar with real curls would ever do—unless, that is, he had an amazing trick to undo the mess he was creating.

When he was done rinsing, he went to get the comb. He returned with a standard fine-toothed, black plastic comb. Now I was nervous. No one who knew how to comb truly curly hair would attempt to comb curls like mine with that weakling comb. But, he announced, it was finally time for his trick! He told me how he'd comb his friend's hair under running water, and the comb would glide right through.

He put my head under the running water, inserted the comb at my hairline, and tugged. The comb didn't budge. The teeth stuck where they were as if my hair were made of tar. He yanked again, but still the comb held tight. Then he froze. At that instant, it must have hit him that my hair wasn't like his friend's hair at all. After a few awkward moments, I said, "It's okay. I'll comb it later." He looked relieved and then untangled his comb from my hair.

I learned a big lesson that day. I learned that people with straight hair, even hairdressers, often think extremely curly hair is like slightly curly hair—just more so. It's not. They are two entirely separate entities, and they must be treated completely differently. That this Santa Cruz hairdresser was certain he knew what to do with very curly hair, even though it quickly became obvious he didn't, is a perfect example of this mindset. Books and experts will say their methods also work for extremely curly hair, but they don't. If it works for straight hair (apart from the standard advice of not damaging it with heat and chemicals), then it most likely doesn't work for our curly hair. Our hair must be treated in almost the opposite way.

I also learned that the only person anywhere around who would know how to comb my hair would have to be me. So ultimately, it's up to you to learn how to comb and protect your hair.

Almost anywhere you go, whether to salons for women of color or not, the main goal of most professionals will be to get you in and out of their chairs as fast as possible, even if that means ripping a comb through your hair in record time. Their interest is in time, not your hair, and certainly not your nerve endings. They will tear through your curls at lightning speed, pulling your hair from its roots, and then joke about how "tender headed" you are (meaning that you still have functioning nerve endings).

When I was a teenager, combing my hair was an ongoing burden. There didn't seem to be a right way to do it. I had no idea what my hair wanted. It was obviously unhappy, but apart from that, I was clueless, and so seemed everyone else. Combing was painful and frustrating every time.

Growing out the part of my hair that was damaged by caustic chemicals and learning an entirely new approach to treating my hair means that it no longer hurts when I comb. Knowing a healthier way to comb my hair means that I don't damage it any longer. With the following techniques, combing will become an opportunity for you to refresh your curls, and a time to create and enjoy each and every quirky new coil.

It will probably be best to first read this whole chapter through, before trying out the techniques. This way you'll know why I make the suggestions I do, and you'll be able to incorporate the ones you like or need into your combing routine. You can also check out the step-by-step photos at the end of this chapter to help clarify any of the following steps.

Comb When Wet, Caution When Dry

Learning how to properly comb your hair will create perfect spirals instead of a big damaged puff that you have to find creative ways to hide. Displaying the beautiful texture of your hair when it's fully expanded and

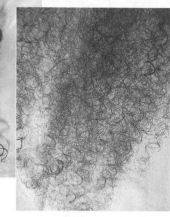

Three dry
curls before
combing . . .

. . . and the same curls after
dry combing.

frizzy is a stunning style with lots of impact. I will sometimes, ever-so-gently, finger-separate my hair to make it big and fuzzy (you can check out my hair like this in chapter 13). What I'm saying is that dry brushing or combing your hair the wrong way *will* damage it severely and limit what you'll be able to do with your hair in the future because of that damage.

First, there are a few rules for our curls. To keep your hair happy and strong and to grow it to its maximum length, it's crucial that you cause as little damage as possible when you comb. Your hair should be combed *only* after washing and conditioning. And then, *only* with the help of a good, slippery conditioner in it. After it's combed and is drying—or dry—it should never be combed (and never, *ever* brushed with a regular brush) again until it has been washed and conditioned again. Combing your curls when they're dry will only make them explode into frizz. And in doing

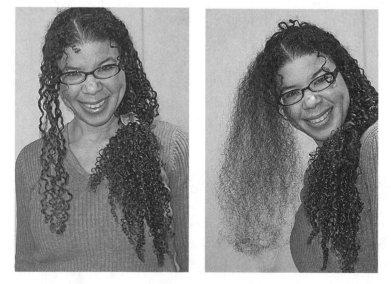

This is what my
hair looks like
when I've combed
it wet with condi-
tioner, defined the
curls, and allowed
them to dry on
their own.

This is what
my hair turns
into if I comb,
brush, or finger-
comb it dry.

so, you'll either break your comb or cause your brush to become hopelessly tangled in the web of fuzz you've created by combing the curls that way.

The rest of this chapter is divided into two parts. The first part is the best way to approach combing to make it as stress-free as possible. The second half covers the actual techniques to make combing as painless and productive as possible.

Note: I use *combing* and *brushing* interchangeably during this chapter, but both terms refer to using a Denman-style brush.

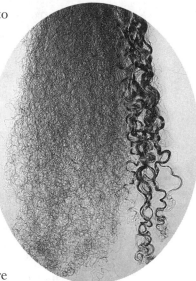

The contrast between before (right) and after (left) I comb my curls dry.

You wouldn't think so, but there's a lot to say about combing. Combing is one of the major hair-care tasks that's most frustrating for us. And this is also where the bulk of the damage occurs to our hair (second to the use of heat and chemicals, that is). Because of this danger, I have so much to tell you about what I've discovered—tips that make combing much easier and no longer damaging. I'll describe each step in more detail as we go along, in case one of these steps gives you trouble with your own hair (or when you comb your child's hair).

First, I'll talk about the best way to approach your hair when you comb it. The attitude you take with your hair can make all the difference in the world in your combing experience. (As I've found out, almost any situation can be a heaven or a hell, depending on how you view it.) Second, I'll get to the basics you need to know to comb your hair without hurting yourself or your hair. I'll talk about prepping your hair to make overall combing easier, what type of comb to use, and how to divide your hair and hold it so that there's no pain when you do comb. I'll also go over the best way to comb it. And finally, I'll give you tips for getting through the challenging spots, like knots and tight mats.

What You Need to Comb Your Hair
- Time to dry your hair. It's best to do this in the morning so that you have the rest of the day to let it dry while you do errands.

- A strong nylon brush with smooth teeth and a rubber base.
- An old pajama top or bathrobe (or any other clothing that you don't mind getting wet with conditioner).
- Soaking-wet hair slathered in conditioner (see chapter 11 for the best ones to use).
- A smooth hair clip to hold back your hair.
- A small pair of sharp scissors to snip off little knots and snarls.
- A smooth barrette or two or a headband to keep the hair off your face while it's drying (this is optional).

You could comb your hair with a wide-toothed comb, but the nicest results are created with a strong styling brush. The best type of brush has a rubber cushion and about nine rows of smooth nylon pins. My favorite is a Denman brush, one of the "Classic Styling Brushes," #D4 (see chapter 11).

Make certain that whatever brush you use, the teeth are *smooth*. Very curly hair will wrap around any little balls at the tips of a comb or a brush and then tangle itself into the brush. You'll have to spend many frustrated minutes extracting the brush from your hair (which happened repeatedly to me until I figured out that brushes with little balls on the tips were not for my curls).

Denman Brushes

Denman is a UK company, but the brushes are usually available at Sally's stores, at other beauty supply stores, and even on Amazon.com. You can go to www.denmanbrush.com to order one or to find more store locations in your area and even to see what the brushes look like. I recommend that you use the Denman D3 or D4 brush.

Make sure that your comb or brush is designed to hold up to your high-spirited hair. It will be worth the investment. I like Denman-type brushes with rubber cushions because they have some give, instead of the give having to come from my hair. Super-curly hair is strong en masse, but your individual strands are fine, so they are easily stretched and hurt. Combing with an unforgiving comb can repeatedly damage your hair by stretching it past its recovery point (see chapter 2). I've also found that regular combs separate everything into an unevenly organized mass, while a regular bristle brush would be ineffective at working through your tangles at best or would get totally wrapped up in your hair at worst. The rows of teeth in a Denman-style brush lock your strands together into curls. Curls hold all of your individual hairs into curl units, which then keep them from puffing.

A New Philosophy for Your Tangles

I love walking. There's a beautiful, overgrown shortcut near my mom's house in Kentucky that I like to take to the store when I'm down visiting her. On my most recent visit, I didn't realize how overgrown the shortcut had become. As I walked, I darted into the undergrowth in the approximate spot I remembered the path to be. I think I had images of being a mysterious woodland creature who could disappear into the tall plants, and no one would be sure whether they'd seen her or their eyes were playing tricks on them.

Well, my version turned out a bit differently. No sooner had I darted into the undergrowth than my hair caught fast and tight in the bushes. It seemed to have instantly wrapped itself into three plants at once, in multiple directions. There went my image of being mysterious. I struggled for long, embarrassing minutes to unwrap my curls from the branches, only to find that more curls had tangled into the plants behind me. It was almost as if I were an insect caught in a spider's web. Luckily, the plants weren't carnivorous. I ended up having to tear myself free. I know there are still hairs of mine wrapped around several branches, hidden within the underbrush of the shortcut.

It makes sense to accept that it's in your curls' very nature to tangle. You can then devote your energy to finding the most constructive way to comb your curls instead of fighting against them. This shift in attitude will make an enormous difference in the relationship you have with your hair.

Set a Time and Accept It: The Zen of Hair Combing

Our hair is not easy to comb. It will tangle. Our spirals and coils are affectionate—they clump and cling to one another. It's a fact, and we must make peace with this in order to work with our hair. There's nothing wrong with our hair because it tangles as it does. Hair that a comb can glide through means that it has no backbone, no fight in it. Because our hair tangles, it takes a certain amount of time to get a comb through it. Mine takes two hours, once a week, to comb. Then I'm done. I accept these two hours and plan for them. I'll watch a movie or television and drink yummy chai tea while I comb. Because I know it takes two hours for me, after forty-five minutes of combing I don't get angry or impatient with my hair because it's "taking so long." I know I still have lots more time left, and I keep working through it carefully and methodically.

It's not a race. If I didn't plan on two hours, then after one hour of working on my hair, I'd have the old loop playing in my head about how it isn't fair. That I *should* be able to get a comb through it like everyone else. I'd be imagining all of the times I've seen people running combs through their straighter hair without incident, and contrasting those mental images with my trying to work out endless tangles, bit by bit. But what good would that do me? The truth is that I do not have straight hair. And many straight-haired people spend good chunks of time and money trying to get body and waves put into theirs.

Combing by Ear: The Curl Whisperer

Combing your hair shouldn't end up sounding like the sound track to a horror film. Tearing, ripping, and snapping sounds, along with hissing or swearing in pain, don't have to be part of your combing routine. Combing can be a quiet and calm process, with the only sound being that of the Denman-type brush softly passing through your hair. Any other sounds mean that something is going wrong. Your ears will serve as your primary defense, giving instant feedback on whether you're simply combing your hair or traumatizing it.

There was a time in my teenage past when people in another part of the house could hear me brushing angrily through my hair. If you hear any tearing, ripping, or snapping sounds while you learn the following techniques, stop immediately. Put down the comb and explore with your fingers. Find out what's going on. If you hear unhappy hair noises while combing, you might be combing over a snarl. And you'll make it worse by doing so, not better. Soon you'll recognize the sound of healthy combing, as well as know instantly when damage is occurring, simply by listening.

Clearing a Path

It helps to have an image in mind of what's happening with your tangles. If you have a game plan, you'll be able to figure out what approach to take when clearing out a tangle. Otherwise, combing is a chaotic, frustrating process, and the goal becomes a rush to rip through your hair as quickly as possible.

The most constructive way I've found to view tangles and plan to get them out is to imagine that they're solid objects that need to be moved through a heavily wooded path. You have to clear the path before an object can make its way through. If the path isn't clear, then the tangle you try to move out will only jam into the other tangles blocking its exit. This will create a tangle-jam. If an entire section is tangled, as it usually will be—this is in the nature of our curls—start from the ends and clear an opening path. From there, you'll move out tangles inch by inch, one by one.

Start by combing your ends. Then move up a little, comb the next tangled section out to the ends, and imagine releasing the tangle from the ends of your hair. Now that the path has been cleared, go up a little farther in the section. Comb this tangle down to the path and out the ends. Make your way up the section. All the while, use the Pinch Grip and the Twist Pinch from the "Pain-Free Combing" section later in this chapter to keep this from hurting.

Beads on a String

Your genes traded ease of combing for volume and your rich hair texture. You simply can't run a comb from the top of your hair to the bottom in one swift motion. This is a property of curly hair. Instead, it's best to move your comb in overlapping steps, to slide your tangles out like pearls on a string.

If your hair is long, you can remove tangles in stages. This is like sliding all the pearls from the top of a long string to the middle, and then moving them from the middle out to the ends. This saves you the effort of moving every bead from the very top to the bottom, one by one.

First, make sure that you've combed out the immediate area where the tangles will be moved into. Move tangles down from your scalp to the middle of the section of hair you're working on, one by one. Then work tangles from the middle out to the ends, sliding them off the bottom, one by one. You're finished with a section when you move out that last tangle. For very curly hair, the difference between combed and not yet combed will be obvious. Hair combed with conditioner is slick and smooth, while hair yet to be combed will be puffy or snarled.

Imagine removing each tangle as if you were removing pearls from a string, one by one.

The tangle is moved down the section of hair like a bead on a string. The ends are combed out, and then the tangle is moved to the ends in stages. Here the tangle has been combed halfway down, and the ends are combed out to give it a place to move into.

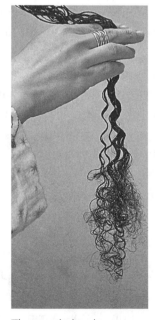

The tangle has been combed into the "empty" spot.

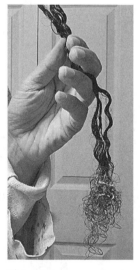

The ends are combed out again, and the final piece of tangle is combed out the ends, like removing the last bead on a string.

How to Keep Combing from Hurting

Pain is your body's way of telling you something is wrong. If combing hurts you or your child, it means you are not combing the right way. *Combing doesn't have to hurt.* When my mom broke her leg, she had to spend some time in the hospital while she recovered. She wasn't able to take care of her hair while she was there, and nurses washed it for her. They washed it the way you see straight-haired people do it in commercials. My mom's hair got so tangled, she couldn't get a comb through it. Often the nurses washed her hair at night, so she ended up sleeping on her wet hair. By the time her leg recovered, her hair was so densely matted, she couldn't get a comb through it at all. In frustration, she hacked off what she could with scissors.

When I was finally able to visit my poor mom, I used the following techniques to work through what remained of her hair-mat. It's to her credit as much as it is to these techniques of preventing pain while combing that she didn't ouch or hiss once during the entire time I combed out her hair.

The following two ways of holding your hair will keep combing from hurting you (or your child): the Pinch Grip and the Twist Pinch.

The Pinch Grip

When you hold the section you're combing, tightly grip your hair between your thumb and index finger. Any tugging is halted at this juncture. This pinch basically seals off the wire transmission your hair is sending and stops it from traveling to the nerve ending in your scalp. You might have to press your fingers together pretty tightly, all the while combing gently. You can also squeeze your hair between your ring finger and center finger for extra protection. Remember, just because it isn't hurting anymore doesn't mean it's okay to comb your hair roughly. It can still be damaged through rough treatment.

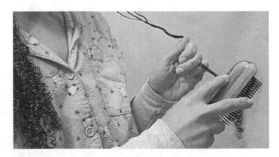

The Pinch Grip seals off the part of your hair you're working on from your sensitive scalp.

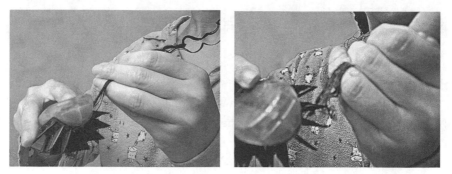

The Pinch Grip. I'm holding my hair firmly between my thumb and index finger. Often, I will also hold it between two additional fingers just to make sure no pain occurs.

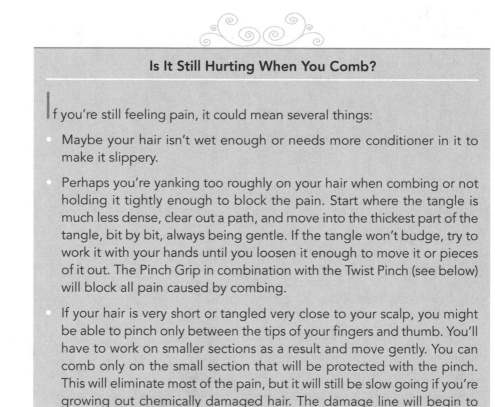

Is It Still Hurting When You Comb?

If you're still feeling pain, it could mean several things:

- Maybe your hair isn't wet enough or needs more conditioner in it to make it slippery.

- Perhaps you're yanking too roughly on your hair when combing or not holding it tightly enough to block the pain. Start where the tangle is much less dense, clear out a path, and move into the thickest part of the tangle, bit by bit, always being gentle. If the tangle won't budge, try to work it with your hands until you loosen it enough to move it or pieces of it out. The Pinch Grip in combination with the Twist Pinch (see below) will block all pain caused by combing.

- If your hair is very short or tangled very close to your scalp, you might be able to pinch only between the tips of your fingers and thumb. You'll have to work on smaller sections as a result and move gently. You can comb only on the small section that will be protected with the pinch. This will eliminate most of the pain, but it will still be slow going if you're growing out chemically damaged hair. The damage line will begin to move down your head as your hair grows out, and it will gradually reveal more glossy new growth that will be easier to comb.

Using the Pinch Grip will become so second nature to you, you'll automatically hold your hair this way when combing it. It's very simple to do and will save you or your child gallons of suffering.

The Twist Pinch

The Twist Pinch is one more safeguard to keep you from hurting yourself when combing your hair. It's another tool in your combing toolbox that helps block pain. If you're working on a matted area of hair, in particular, you'll need to use this technique.

While combing, simply twist the section you're working on anywhere between your scalp and the combing area. You'll usually need to give it only one turn. If you're in a snarled spot, two or three turns should be plenty. Then use the Pinch Grip to seal it off while you comb.

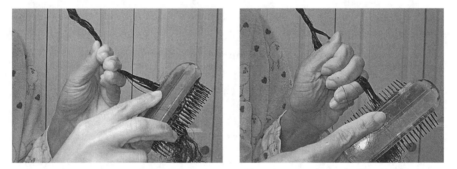

Twisting your hair and pinching it between your fingers keeps it from hurting your scalp when you comb. (In these photos, I'm not combing all the way down to the ends. I'm combing only a few inches of hair, then I'll move in overlapping sections down to the ends.)

Why Comb Wet?

Many books may tell you to avoid brushing your hair when it's wet. This is reasonable for straighter hair, because a comb goes quickly through dry straighter hair within minutes. Or seconds. The big concern with brushing straighter hair when it's wet is to prevent stretching it, thereby damaging it. Wet hair is more vulnerable than dry hair (see chapter 2), so when it's brushed or combed roughly, it's more prone to getting stretched and damaged. When I see people with straighter hair comb their hair, they often do it from the scalp straight down to the ends in a few swift, broad strokes. Even when they start at the bottom of their hair, tangles are simply ripped out from the ends in record time. The presence of a few tangles slows the process by only a few seconds to minutes when combing an entire head of straighter hair. A tangle or two in straighter hair is different from having very curly hair with a head full of nothing but tangles. Yet even though tangles aren't a big deal for people with straighter hair, combing their hair while it's wet and vulnerable will stretch it. It's better to comb straighter hair when it's as dry as possible, to protect it.

For very curly hair, though, combing is an entirely different process. I wouldn't be able to comb my hair at all if I had to comb it dry. Combing super-curly hair when it's dry can be exhausting at best. Combs don't glide through it. In fact, they often get tangled in the hair instead. Your hair gets bigger and bigger as curls are separated, and it becomes an increasing struggle to get through them. The brute force that must be used to get a comb through your hair will not only wear your hair away, but tear it out. Your ends are dry and unprotected, flailing around like little curly tentacles, and they'll snarl fiercely together. It's difficult to reach your scalp through the giant dandelion puff your hair has now become. This turns into such an ordeal, you might be tempted to rip through your hair. While combing your hair dry can do a huge amount of damage, combing your hair by using the techniques in this book will cause little, if any, damage. This is because wet, conditioned curls are slippery, so the comb slides through with less effort than if your hair was dry. Wet curly hair is easier to manage, and, when done properly and with a giving brush, your wet hair doesn't stretch much more when combed wet than dry (remember, I use "combing" and "brushing" interchangeably when referring to using a Denman-type brush). Also, by using the Pinch Grip, what little stretching might occur is isolated to only the spots you're combing at that moment.

With your hair wet and conditioned, it stays manageable as you comb it. It stays clumped together, the brush slips through relatively easily, and tangles will come undone more quickly. The Denman-type brush's rubber cushion absorbs much of the tension caused by any pulling. This means that the give comes from the rubber cushion, rather than from your hair.

Pre-Combing Your Trouble Spots

When combing your hair, there are a few techniques that will make the entire process much easier. These tips will minimize snarling and tangling if you use these precautions before you start combing in earnest. They prepare the canvas of your hair for combing to go as smoothly as possible.

Comb Your Ends First

After you apply the combing conditioner, you need to comb the ends of your hair. This will loosen and prepare them for when the rest of your hair is divided into more manageable pieces. You'll comb the ends of your hair first to clear a path for the rest of your tangles to come out. Combing the ends will also reduce your hair's tangling potential by giving the ends a clean slate, instead of adding newer tangles into older tangles. The rest of the pre-combing tips will help you work out the most tangled spots to make overall combing easier.

Diffuse Very Matted Bits

You'll also want to check whether any lumpy matted areas are lurking in your hair. Sometimes the hair at the back of your neck may be extra tangled; the same goes for sections that rub against your shirt collar or that get slept on more than other parts. If certain patches feel dense with tangles, it's a good idea to comb these a bit to loosen some of the tangles before you start to comb the rest of your hair. Otherwise, they'll prevent you from pre-combing the hair near your scalp.

Pre-Combing Hair at Your Scalp: A Shortcut

It's sometimes easier to pre-comb hair at your roots first, to prevent worse tangling later when you're nearly done. This is because as you comb from the bottom of your hair up, there's less room for your comb to reach an individual section at the scalp. I often accidentally snag freshly combed hair at my hairline, causing sections I've already finished to tangle up again. This means I have to comb them again, and in doing that, just like pushing over one domino, I end up snarling a different freshly combed section. Therefore, this technique helps you avoid this frustration by pre-combing your hair directly over your scalp. This way, when you comb your way up to the pre-combed section, you know you can stop there. This prevents you from snagging hair that's already been combed.

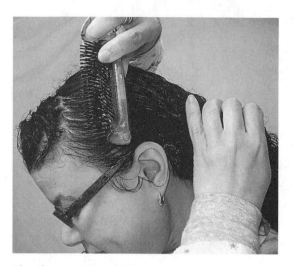

The shortcut: I'm combing my hair at my scalp first, and then I'll start combing from the ends up. Once this area is combed, I don't have to comb it again. You can see that I have conditioner all over me. I have the front part of my hair pinned back because I have such a low hairline. I do that area separately.

To try this shortcut, start near the back of your head and comb only the hair closest to your scalp in the direction it grows. Move to the area above your ears, then to the crown. The brush or the comb needs to smooth only the hair at your scalp. When you're done with the first half, clip it back, and do the same on the other half of your hair. Later, as you're combing each section from the bottom up, you'll meet up with this pre-combed part. When that happens, you're finished!

Exception to the Shortcut

I can do this shortcut because my roots are much straighter than the rest of my hair is, but the shortcut isn't really necessary. In fact, if your hair is very tangled or matted, such as when you are first growing out a perm, you should not do this step. Your mats could be so tightly crammed together that pre-combing your scalp area might actually jam them more tightly together. In that case, it's best to start at your ends and work up to these mats. This way, you'll have cleared a path for the mats to move out of your hair.

Getting Your Hair into Bite-Size Pieces

After pre-combing any troubled spots, the best way to tackle combing very thick hair is to divide and conquer. As always, your first priority is keeping your ends as calm and smooth as possible. This prevents them from snarling up.

You'll start by dividing your wet, conditioned hair in half. You can put it into two loose buns or separate it with clips. This keeps the section you aren't working on out of your way. Your hair doesn't have to be perfectly divided in half. Divide your hair the way it wants to be divided. Sometimes it might end up being in three sections, or one half might end up being much bigger than the other half. It's all good. Because your hair hasn't been combed, it'll want to cling to itself. If the two sections of your hair don't separate easily (without any tearing noises), clip as much as you can of the half you *won't* be working on out of your way. As you finish combing one side, you'll meet with the other half in the middle anyway. Then you'll have another shot at gently dividing the two halves.

To Divide into Smaller Working Sections

Undo one side of your hair. Hold it in the Pinch Grip between your thumb and index finger or in your fist, to keep it from being yanked when you comb. Comb out all of the ends in that chunk of hair. By brushing your ends first, you reduce your hair's tendency to snarl as you begin to divide it into smaller, more manageable pieces.

When your ends are combed, gently separate out a small section of hair, about an inch wide, that you'll be able to easily work with. The size of the section depends on how tight your curls are or how long or tangled your hair is. Tightly curled or tangled hair needs to be divided into smaller, more easily managed sections. Average sections should be about one inch square to start with. Never yank your hair apart. Never separate sections by dividing your hair like a wishbone. When you start at the top of a section and pull it apart, your ends will spin and snare tighter and tighter together, until they lock in a death grip and have to be cut out. As soon

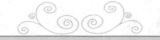

Is Separating Sections Still Difficult?

If separating your hair into sections for combing gives you trouble, several things might be causing this:

- Your hair might need more conditioner or water and conditioner if it's drying out. Have a spray bottle filled with water nearby. It's the wet conditioner that helps make your hair slippery.

- Your hair might need to be combed more often (always while wet with conditioner, of course) if it's taking longer than two hours to comb it each time. Try every four days if you've been going once a week.

- Securing your hair more firmly at night before you sleep will also help reduce tangles. (Never pull your hair so tight that it hurts, however, because it will cause breakage.) When I was growing out my relaxer, I'd get solid mats near my hairline where the chemical section met the new growth when I slept on it. I learned to secure that area firmly until the chemical-damaged sections grew out farther. It still matted until I cut off the damaged hair, but not as tightly.

as you encounter any resistance, *stop* and comb out the ends again or untangle with your fingers. Conditioner helps make your hair slippery, but your hair can still snarl faster than the speed of sound.

There's a trick to separating your hair: Hold the ends of both sections you'd like to separate in one hand. Hold them as if you're asking someone to draw straws. Now with your other hand, slowly ease out one section from the other. Pull it slowly up and away from the rest of the hair, as if you're now drawing out that straw from your own hand. All the while that you're pulling your hair out, hold loosely onto the remaining ends to keep them from snarling. Let the moving section slide through your fingers. If it snarls or makes tearing sounds, stop and comb it or finger-comb. It's okay to comb out the ends again, this time combing a bit higher up the section. Comb your ends as many times as you need to get the job done. Use this technique any time you need to pull your hair apart.

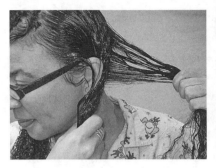

I divide my hair gently, until it starts
to get stuck.

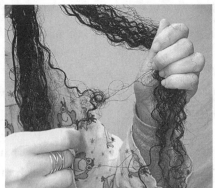

It's in my hair's
nature to tangle.
To pull it apart
without it snarling,
I loosely hold one
section in one hand
and gently pull the
section I want out
of it. Make sure
your hair is wet
with conditioner so
that it's slippery.

Again, never pull your sections apart from the scalp down to the ends
like a wishbone. I keep saying this because you'll want to do it. I do.
I know better, but I get lazy and sometimes try to pull two sections apart.
I always end up having to get the scissors.

Ease your sections apart by holding the ends. Keep eagle eyes
on those ends! If they get
a chance, they'll try to
tangle. They can't help
themselves.

Armed with these tools,
it's time to comb.

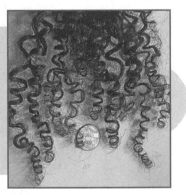

My roots look
straight because the
weight of my wet hair plus
the conditioner weighs them
down. My ends are very tightly
curled (here are my end curls
with a penny for size
comparison).

Ready to Comb

Never underestimate the power of your hair's tangling ability. When I try
on clothes in a hurry, sometimes I forget to put my hair back into a bun.
I'll pull off a shirt, and right when both of my hands are in the air, with the
shirt over my head, I realize with a yank that I'm caught. My hair wraps
around buttons, and I don't realize it's happened at first because it takes
some distance before the spiral uncoils enough for me to feel the tug. It's
not the most graceful sight when I work the shirt back over my head.

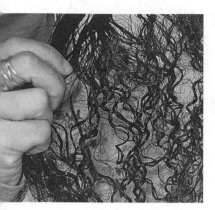

My hair before combing is a network of tangles.

Once my hair has claimed the shirt, just to make it interesting it grabs a few more buttons while I'm freeing all of us.

These suggestions might seem like I'm telling you to pack four suitcases for a weekend trip, but you'll need all of them (the suggestions, but probably not so many suitcases). Maybe you won't use all of these tips at one time, but I use most of them every time I comb my hair. And I've used them *all* at some point. If you have hair like mine, you might end up being really glad for all four tips. These tips can turn chaos into order. I no longer end up with a sore head when I'm done.

That being said, make sure your hair is very wet and drenched with conditioner. Start at the back of your head. This will make it easier to clip finished sections out of the way, to the other side, when you're done.

Loosen a manageable chunk of hair to tackle, carefully separating it from the herd by using the sectioning tips mentioned earlier in this chapter. When the piece you want to work on is separated, clip the rest of the section out of your way.

As always, start with the very ends of your hair and gently comb out the tips before you move up the section. This clears a path for tangles to move into. If necessary, detangle clumps with your fingers and then try to comb that section through again. Always hold your working section in a Pinch Grip or a Twist Pinch, *above* the spot you're combing.

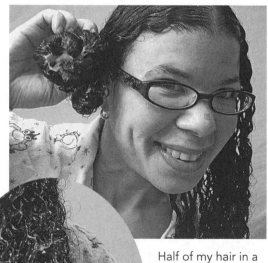

Half of my hair in a bun (above), the other half down and ready to be divided for combing (left). You can see how much conditioner is in the bun and the section I'm about to comb.

Start combing below the tangle and work your way up. In particularly snarled spots, you might have to divide the section again. Use as your guide the pieces that seem to naturally want to separate from the rest or sections that can be easily pulled from the rest. The smaller you can make the tangled spot, the easier it'll be to get through.

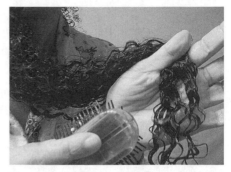

I comb my ends first. This makes dividing out a manageable section easier.

Move up about two inches and comb down to the ends again. Remember, this is like moving pearls off a string, one by one. If your hair isn't tightly curled or not too tangled, you can move up several inches at a time. Very tangly or very tightly curled hair needs to be combed in smaller steps.

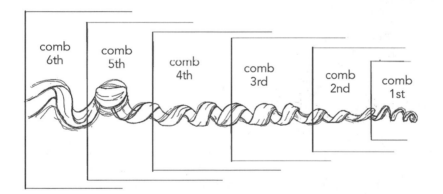

comb 6th   comb 5th   comb 4th   comb 3rd   comb 2nd   comb 1st

The basic order of combing your curls.

By working in sections, you'll ensure that your ends are always tended to. If you don't pay attention, those ends will snarl as quickly as a fly will land on your food when you look away. When you make it to your scalp (or the pre-combed area at the scalp) and ease the last tangle from your ends, you're done with that section.

When you've finished a section and removed every tangle, it's not necessary to do a final combing from scalp to ends. This stretches your hair unnecessarily—not to mention that you could potentially catch on the parts you've already combed and snag them. Your hair is thoroughly combed when it's been combed in overlapping sections. I've found that if I try to run a comb from my scalp to the ends, I *never* make it to the ends. My hair always snarls somewhere. By combing in overlapping steps, I know that each overlapping segment is tangle free, which means the entire section will be tangle free once I reach the bottom.

Step-by-Step Photo Guide to Combing Your Hair

This shows all of the steps in combing very curly hair. The entire process takes only about two hours, once a week, and then you will have easy-to-care-for hair the rest of the week.

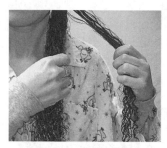

I now have a manageable section to work with.

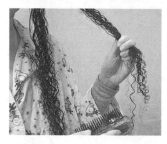

I'm ready to start combing. The ends are beginning to dry out. I spritz them with water to get them damp again. Also, don't be afraid to add more conditioner. You can see I still had some in my brush.

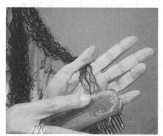

I comb the ends, holding my hair in a pinch between my thumb and forefinger to keep the pressure I use from hurting my scalp.

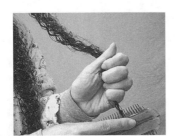

I work my way up the ends. In really tangled spots, I grip my hair tightly so that it doesn't pull at my scalp. This also prevents me from stretching the entire section of hair when I comb.

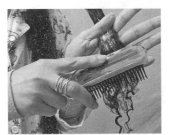

I've worked my way up to the pre-combed area at my scalp. From there, I move down and comb out the last tangles. I keep combing the tangle down my hair. I comb pieces of the tangle out from the bottom, then down into the newly cleared spot.

The tangle inches down my hair. I keep combing it out by combing away the bottom of the tangle, then moving the tangle closer to the ends. I move the tangle from my hair like a bead from a necklace.

Here I'm combing out the bottom of the tangle.

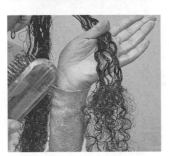

Now I'm inching the rest of the tangle into the newly cleared spot. You can really see the difference between my combed and uncombed hair.

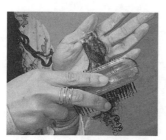

The tangle is moved to the ends. Notice how foamy the conditioner is.

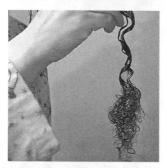

The tangles have been moved out of my hair, leaving the last tangle to be removed. Again, you can see the difference that combing with conditioner makes, when you compare my combed and uncombed curls.

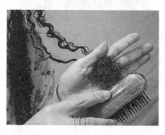

To remove the tangle, I comb out the ends so that the tangle has a spot to move into. Then I'll comb the tangle down into the cleared spot.

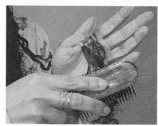

I comb the tangle down farther toward the ends. You can see all of the conditioner on my hand.

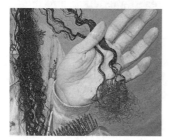

Then the tangle teeters at the ends of my hair.

Sometimes your ends really foam up, and other times the conditioner is combed into your hair by the time you're through. Either way is fine, as long as there's still plenty of conditioner in your hair by the time you're done. The foamy conditioner will disappear by the time you separate and smooth your curls. The conditioner also loosens my curls. My ends are actually very tightly curled, but when wet with conditioner, they loosen enough to let me comb them.

Remember, combing doesn't have to hurt. Learning these techniques and being patient while you use them will prevent pain. Your hair is helpless. Be kind to it and learn to care for it, instead of abusing it, and you'll soon have longer, *healthy* hair.

> ### Condition in Comfort
>
> Conditioner can drip everywhere, so it doesn't hurt to wear some comfy pajamas when you comb. You could even put a towel down to protect your furniture.

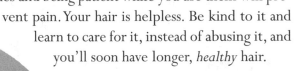

Done! The conditioner will foam up as you comb through your hair. This is actually a good thing. It means you're using enough. Don't worry—it disappears by the time you smooth your curls in the next step.

> ### Embrace Your Foam
>
> Know that as you comb, the conditioner will foam up in your hair as if your hair has gone rabid. This is normal. By the time you finish combing and separating your curls, the conditioner will vanish. Actually, seeing the foam is a good thing. It means you've used enough conditioner. And don't worry; if for some reason there's still a little conditioner left when you're done, simply dab the spot with water and pat with a towel, and it's gone.

Challenges

When combing your hair, it's best to have some tricks ready in case you run into some very tangled spots. These will help guide you through any snarls, knots, and mats you might run across, and help you to minimize any damage from occurring when you remove them.

Snip It, Don't Rip It

With curly hair, your ends knot up no matter how carefully you treat them. You can use scissors for small, tight snarls and knots near the ends. It's no big deal. With curly hair, a tiny snip at the ends won't show in the least. When the ends are cut, it's a clean cut, and the rest of your hair shaft

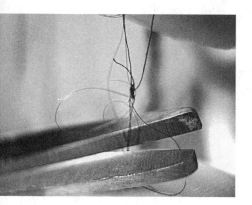

It's better to snip out a tangle than to risk stretching those hairs and damaging them by trying to pull the tangle out.

is undamaged. If you rip a tangle out of your hair, however, it stretches your hair, usually beyond its limits. Afterward, the strands of hair involved in the snarl-pulling are now damaged and weakened, and they don't recover. It's far better to remove the snarl with a little snip, leaving the remaining hair undamaged.

Snipping is fine for tiny bits of hair, fewer than about twenty strands. The snarl or the knot should be no bigger than a bead. A knot this tiny is nearly impossible to undo, especially a tight one. I keep a small pair of scissors next to me when I comb, to cut off all the knots and the snarls I encounter. I end up having to snip off at least two little snarls every time I comb.

If the knot is larger, you could try to undo it as you would a piece of knotted thread, or try to slide as much hair out from it as possible. Do this by first locating the core of the knot and then finding the hairs not directly involved in the knot. Often, only a few hairs will knot together and hold a bunch of other hairs hostage. Try to free these "hostage hairs" before you cut the truly locked ones. This is best done by loosely holding the knot in one hand and gently sliding hairs out of it with the other hand. The conditioner makes it slippery enough that hairs might glide loose if they aren't directly involved. If there's resistance, stop at once and untangle with your fingers. If the snarl is huge, try to lightly comb the ends. Sometimes this helps release hairs that are not directly tangled. If it makes tearing sounds, stop. If none of the hairs in the knot wants to budge, just cut the tangle out. It won't show, and there isn't much else you can do but minimize damage.

Little Dot Knots

Because our hairs are twisty and fine, individual strands sometimes tie themselves into knots. They feel like the tiniest beads stuck to your hair. Up close, you can see they are knots, exactly like the ones tied on a string. Just cut them off if you feel like it. I usually do this when I'm combing. If I run into several of them clustered at the end of a curl, I give the end a little snip, and they're gone. If you have these dot knots, you didn't do anything wrong to cause them. It just happens with super-curly hair.

Mats

Mats shouldn't happen very often if you treat your hair in a soothing way. They do occur ferociously, however, when you're growing out a relaxer, usually at the border between your new growth and the chemically processed hair. Other things that can cause matting are sleeping on your hair when it's wet and not well secured, and sleeping on puffy hair without securing it firmly. Mats frequently occur near the scalp, where they are not only difficult to reach but can really hurt if you're not extremely careful.

When I was growing out my relaxer, my chemically damaged hair reached to about my shoulders before it shattered into thousands of pieces and grew no farther. During the growing-out period, I set it in many two-strand twists. It took me three hours every week to get a comb through my shoulder-length hair and twist it into about twenty twists. Each week I got tight mats where my old chemically damaged hair met the new growth. The mats snuggled in close to the back of my head and hurt like anything to get out of my hair. Because they pressed themselves right against my head, I had no way to comb them without it hurting. There wasn't enough room to use any Pinch Grips. Luckily, this lasted only a few months, until my hair grew out enough that I could pinch above the mat to keep it from hurting my scalp.

If possible, try to isolate the mat you're working on. Move any hair that's near it out of the way. Make sure the mat has conditioner on it, and work more conditioner into it by gently poking into it with your fingers and squeezing it. Try to carefully ease out any hairs that aren't tightly tangled into the mat. Ease the mat apart if possible. To do this, you'll need to burrow a finger into the mat and move it around to make the hole bigger. Then put a couple more fingers into it, enough to try to gently pry it apart. See whether you can divide it. It might be willing to be broken into several smaller mats that you can tackle one by one.

Clear a pathway for the mat by combing your ends. Comb up your hair in overlapping steps until you reach the bottom of the mat. Gently take little "nibbles" off the mat by combing its outer edges. Sometimes you'll be able to comb your way into the heart of a mat, and then it usually breaks apart into smaller pieces. When you can separate a section from the main mat, comb it down and out of your hair. Then return, loosen more of the mat from the bottom, and comb that out, chipping away until it's gone.

Very tight mats might be so firm that you can't even get the nylon pins of the comb into them. In extreme cases, start at the base of the mat, always making sure a path has been cleared for it first. Take your brush and lightly, softly, stroke the bottom edge of the mat. This can loosen bits of hair off the mat, enough to slide them out from the main mat body. Tight mats take *lots* of patience. Keep brushing ever so gently at the mat's base to loosen more hair. The more hair you can get out of the mat, the smaller it becomes. Try to separate even the smallest pieces possible from it. Work at loosening the mat with your fingers again. Scavenge from the mat; take away any hair you can get from it.

If your entire head is matted, the combing principles are still the same. It will take more work, though. Use lots of conditioner to keep your hair slippery, and ease apart whatever you can off the main mat. You can't be choosy at this point. Any bit of hair you can set free from the main body of the mat is good. Comb this small bit, pin it safely out of the way, and return for more. Work your way through each mat. This is more a question of will than anything else. If you have enough patience and stamina, you can get through an entire matted head. I know; I've done it way too many times in my youth.

Things to Keep Your Eagle Eyes On

You might also run across more serious problems happening with the ends of your hair. Your ends are active, so it's good to check in on them. I always give a few randomly selected curls an exam when I comb my hair.

You might run into some split ends or breakage. Always cut these off. Finding them occasionally is normal. If most of the ends of your hair are broken or splitting, however, you should get them all cut off. This is more serious, because it is a sign that damage has happened or is still happening. Using the techniques in this book won't cause damage, so in time you'll see very few split ends and little breakage. But if you're just starting, you'll have to deal with residual damage from previous techniques until the damaged parts are gone.

What's Left

Our head sheds about 100 to 150 hairs a day (see chapter 2). If you normally comb your hair every day, you get used to seeing this amount of hair in your comb. When you begin to comb your hair once a week, you might have 700 to 1,050 hairs in your comb. The wad of hair you pull from your comb will appear to be the size of a very tangled mouse. This is normal. If, however, you suddenly begin to pull hair off your comb that amounts to the size of, say, a guinea pig, you might want to check with a doctor to make sure everything is okay.

It's important to understand that combing your hair isn't a race. You might win the struggle to get a comb through your hair in record time, but in doing so you'll ultimately lose when you end up with shredded hair

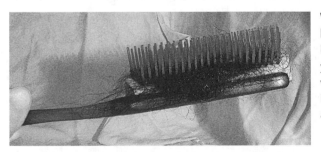

What's left in the brush. It looks like lots of hair, but you're seeing a week's worth at once instead of a little at a time.

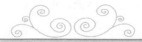

Money-Saving Tip

You can finally use up those shampoos you don't really like to clean your Denman-style brush. After combing your hair, fill the sink with a couple inches of warm water. Remove the hair from the brush and submerge the brush in the water. Squirt shampoo over the rubber base, flip it over, and swish it around in the water for a minute. When the shampoo has dissolved into the sink water, rinse the brush in warm water. Then hang your brush up to dry for the next time.

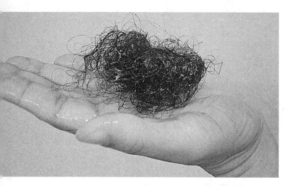

My pet fuzz ball. It's up to you whether you throw it out or use it to stuff beaded purses (or, hey, even stuffed animals).

that breaks off at your shoulders and grows no farther. Most of all, we lose when we direct our impatience and anger toward something that's a part of us. Learning to accept and work with your hair's tangled nature will reward you with pain-free, peaceful combing, and long, gleaming spirals.

When you finish combing each section of hair, you'll set your curls before pinning them up and moving on to the next section to comb. The next chapter describes how to reinforce and weatherproof your curls to prevent frizz, giving you worry-free hair.

I'm not able to run my hands through my hair, so I need to separate my curls out one by one. If you can't run your fingers through your hair either, the next chapter, which explains how to define your curls, is for you. If you're able to run your fingers through your hair, you can skip the next chapter and simply run your fingers through your hair from scalp to ends, making sure there's plenty of conditioner in it. This will separate and define your curls. (See also "Shortcut, or for Looser Curls" at the end of chapter 6.)

- Our hair tangles. We must accept this reality.

- Because our hair is curly, it takes longer to comb it properly.

- Never separate bunches of your hair like a wishbone.

- Take care of your ends first. Keep your eyes on those rascals at all times.

- Listen to your hair for sounds of trouble—it'll let you know.

- When combing, hold your hair by pinching it between your fingers to prevent painful pulling on your scalp.

- Comb your hair only when it's soaking wet and loaded with conditioner.

- Comb in sections.

- Start from your ends and work up.

- Clear a path, and then move tangles out one by one, like beads on a string.

- When you have a snarl or a knot you can't work out, snip, don't rip.

- Make sure your hair remains soaking wet with water and conditioner. Keep a spray bottle and your conditioner handy.

Chapter Six

Setting Perfect Curls
Born to Clump

Twice in high school, I went to get my hair trimmed at salons that had much less curly clients. At the first salon, after my hair was washed and trimmed, I mentioned that my hair got really fuzzy when it was brushed dry. The stylist gave my hair a few light spritzes with water and began to brush it with vigor. She might have believed that at some point my expanding hair would deflate again with enough brushing, and the curls would all curl back together again with enough persistence. She was wrong. When she was done, I had a giant mushroom head. Easily mortified teenager that I was, I thrust the money at her and ran out of the shop with my hands over my head. I darted into the nearest bathroom and put my head under the faucet to wet down my hair.

The second time I went for a trim, I had a well-meaning adult companion follow me on my dash into the bathroom afterward. She stopped me from putting my head under the faucet. Instead, she tried to helpfully "pick" my hair, thinking perhaps that jabbing large plastic teeth into my giant cloud of hair would somehow put my curls back together again. She told me it would work because she used this pick on her hair (her straight hair that had been curly-permed, that is), and besides, picks were supposed to be for African hair, so, of course, it would work (even though picks are generally used to fluff up very curly hair and separate the curls, not bind them back together again). Finally, she relented and let me put my head under the tap. My hair was in its fully expanded position, and there was nothing that could be done to restore my texturized curls back into curls otherwise.

Do know that I now love the look of my hair when it's fully expanded. There are few styles more stunning. At the time, however, I hated feeling I had no choice about how my hair looked and reacted. This was made worse because I was a shy teenager who only wanted to blend in, and it made me want to turn myself inside out to avoid looking different. Now I love that my hair is unique, and I love its expansive nature. I am also glad I have control over when it's big and when it's curly. Because I have this choice, I can enjoy all of its looks.

What we need to do, to make the most of our curls, is the opposite of what the hairdressers, the magazines, and our well-meaning friends may tell us. Instead of pulling our curls apart through brushing, if we want to display their curly texture, we need to find ways to put our spirals back together again and help them stay that way. This truly showcases each and every beautiful curl we have.

Leave in That Conditioner!

I know this advice sounds radical, and it seems like you'll end up with white gloppy hair by leaving in conditioner. It only starts out gloppy, however, until you comb it in. Thick, natural curls soak up conditioner like sponges when you comb it in. For the conditioner to work, however, you do need to use one with the right ingredients. If you use one that has sticky ingredients in it (see chapter 11), your hair will be crunchy and sticky, and there will be massive buildup.

When I first started to leave conditioner in my hair, I found that the times when I felt I'd put in too much, I got the best results. Although the conditioner looked gluey and white when wet, it didn't dry like that. Conditioner is forgiving and easy to work with. It's difficult to use too much in very curly hair. It gets foamy as you comb, but by the time you're done smoothing each curl, all you'll see is wet hair (see the "Step-by-Step Photo Guide to Combing Your Hair" at the end of chapter 5). Any excess conditioner is combed off by the brush and will most likely be redistributed to sections that need more conditioner. As long as your hair is nice and wet, an oversaturated section of hair simply won't hold the extra amount. The conditioner vanishes by the time your hair is combed, but it's still there, doing its job. If, when your hair is nearly dry, there's a spot that got extra conditioner, it's easy to wet your fingers and dab the spot. Then you can smooth the conditioner back into your hair.

Define Each Curl, and the Weather Won't Matter

In my late teens, I went to the ocean with three friends. This wasn't a balmy tropical ocean, but the cold and windy shores of the Northwest. My friends all had naturally straight hair and came from straight-haired families. At the time I'd just taken out my weave and was still trying to figure out what to do with my hair. At night I was experimenting with brushing out my chin-length hair and sleeping with a bandanna firmly tied over it to press my curls down into waves (see the photo in chapter 1 under "Extensions").

Wearing the bandanna was a huge source of embarrassment. I always tried to hide that bandanna wrap from my blond college roommate. I either snatched it off my head when she walked into the room, as if she'd walked in on me doing something I shouldn't have, or I slept with my blankets over my head so she couldn't see it.

Anyway, that day my friends and I drove down to the ocean and walked along the shore. The wind whipped around ferociously, churning up the waves and pelting us with mist. I felt my hair whipping around and tried to hold my hands over it. It was too short to pull back in any way. We walked for a couple of hours and then went back to the car, where the wind finally quieted. Just as we were about to get into the car, my three friends turned and stared at me with stunned expressions.

"What?" I said, feeling a lump in my stomach.

"Your hair," one of my friends said in disbelief. "It's *huge*. It's in a perfect circle." He drew a round shape around my head with his hand. He wanted to take a picture, but I wouldn't let him. What kept going through my head was, Why can't my hair just act like normal hair for once? I rode the rest of the way back to the dorms scowling, pressing my hair down to my head with both hands.

Now I live in Seattle, and I walk around almost every day in the wind and the rain. I took a good portion of the photographs for this book after I'd walked in just such weather. This should tell you two things: One is that I don't seem to have enough sense to carry an umbrella. The second is that these techniques really do keep your hair from reacting to the weather. The fourth technique to make your hair happy is defining each of your curls to create perfect, weatherproof coils. It will also make it easier to divide your hair later on when you go to style it, because you're pre-dividing each curl now.

Our hair wants to clump. Since all of the strands in a curl have a similar curl pattern, they naturally want to lock together. Brushing while dry and the wind that day at the oceanside forced my hair to separate into individual strands. But when you take each curl and smooth all of the hairs together within it, you're working *with* your hair's clumping nature. After smoothing, each strand of hair is held securely next to its curly neighbor strand. The conditioner helps to reinforce them. Now, each strand of hair in the curl is snuggled like a spoon with other hairs just like it. Your curly hairs are bonded into a tight-spiraled community, where they're safe and surrounded by other curls that share their particular curl pattern. They're supporting one another in a happy curly commune, and they don't want to go anywhere. This makes them resistant to wind and weather because your strands are now acting like *curl units* instead of individual hairs.

When you wet-comb a section of your hair, it begins to divide on its own into curls. If the combed section isn't dividing on its own and looks like an unbroken sheet of hair, shake it gently. This causes your curls to start breaking apart into curl units.

To set and free individual curls, take each curl that's separating in this combed section and, one by one, gently pull it from its neighbor curls. Keep the ends smooth by carefully holding your curls at the bottom, and pull out the curl segment you want. When one little curl section has been freed, run your hand down it in the direction it will be hanging. This smooths and unifies all of the hairs together into one curl.

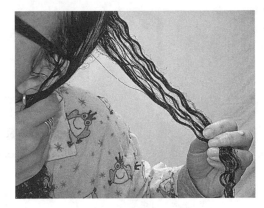

When you comb your hair, it will begin to separate into the curls it would like to have. Divide your combed hair into these curls. If I left my hair like this, the curls would be unfocused and meshed together and would get puffy easily.

After choosing a curl, I divide it from the rest of my hair. Make sure there's enough conditioner to make your curls clump together properly.

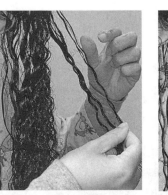
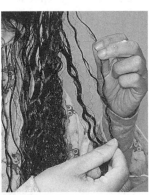
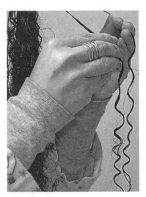

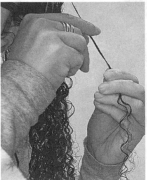
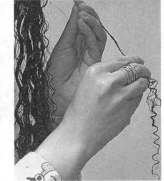

Smooth each segment between your fingers to set them into firm curl units. I run one or both of my fingers down the separated curl to smooth and lock all of the hairs in place. Notice how disorganized the segment in these two photos looks before smoothing. This process lines up all of the hairs into a single curl unit that can withstand the weather. You can see all of the hairs before I smooth them, looking confused.

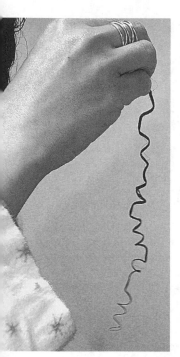

Make sure your curl feels smooth all the way down its length. If there's a rough spot, you can comb the curl smooth. Go over only that curl with your comb, and then run your fingers down it again. If too much hair has been included in one curl, you'll see it popping apart into two or more pieces. It's always best to go with what your curl wants. Try to divide your curls the way they're separating. This lets your curls tell you exactly what they want.

The curliness of your hair will play a large part in the size of these segments. Curlier hair might need more curls to be separated and smoothed per inch than looser curls would. Sometimes the sizes of your curls vary across your head. In some places, more curls will need to be made than in other spots. For me, the top and the back of my head are very curly, and the bottom is somewhat curly (relative to the top). So I end up setting nearly

This is the same curl after being defined. Now all of the hairs in it will act more like one curl unit. They're bonded together, and they're happy this way. They don't want to pouf anymore.

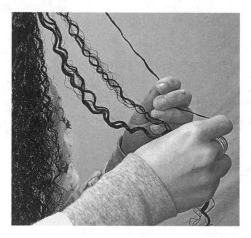

I'm smoothing another curl between my fingers, while holding the rest of my curls that still need to be smoothed in my right hand. I repeat this process of combing a section and then smoothing out the curls.

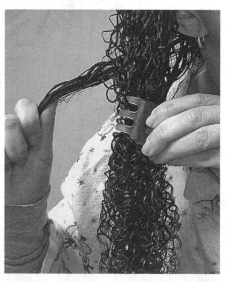

When I finish a section, I clip it back out of the way and move to another section.

twice as many smaller curls on the top and back parts of my head as on the nape of my neck and around my ears.

Defining your hair like this lets all of the individual strands of each curl clump together in the way they want to go. When you comb your hair and don't separate and smooth, your hair behaves like one giant mass. All of your curls are curled together. Parts of one curl will be included in other neighbor curls. A few curls might break free, but the rest will be disorganized. They'll frizz easily because they don't have a direction. Your curls need your help to reinforce them into strong, firm curls.

Curls formed without separating are netted together.

Curls formed after separating are well defined.

The difference between curls combed but not defined and curls after defining.

When I've finished combing and defining my hair, I leave it alone to dry. At first, it looks stringy. This is good. It means I used enough conditioner to do the job, and my curls are setting. When my hair is dry, I pull it back in a bun or a braid and sleep on it. This further calms the curls and stretches them out even more. In the morning, I undo my bun or braid and put my hair in a simple style. All I have to do for the rest of the week is put my hair up each night and smooth a little water and conditioner on it each morning to refresh it, and help my curls spring back into coils.

Before I discovered setting my individual curls, I found it next to impossible to divide my hair to style it. It was meshed together like netting. I spent so many angry hours pulling my hair apart and ended up with expanses of fuzz and snarls afterward. Our hair *does not* like to be pulled apart. By dividing your curls, you're actually pre-separating them. Now each curl is reinforced, and it behaves like one unit instead of being connected to every other curl on your head.

For the best, noncrunchy, nonsticky results, don't use gel or holding products. Conditioner does it all.

For Short Hair: Doodles

My mother has curls as tight as mine. Recently, she has been experimenting with wearing her hair naturally. After her stay in the hospital, once we combed out her hair, she decided to try wearing her hair short.

She uses a variation of what I do to smooth her curls. Because her coils are shorter, there isn't enough hair to run her fingers down the length of every curl. Instead, after washing and leaving conditioner in her hair, she takes individual curls and twists each one around her finger. She calls the cute little spirals doodles. She's gotten lots of compliments on them. They sort of make her curls mini–Shirley Temple curls. This style is also perfect for guys who wear their hair

This is Aja before she combs and sets her hair.

Stunning Aja after she's finished combing and defining all of her curls.

Aja starts out by putting in lots of conditioner and pinning up all of her hair except the section she is about to work on.

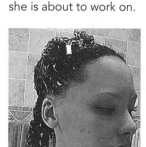

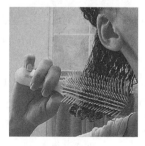

She combs the section she's separated out with a Denman.

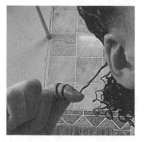

She takes each curl and twirls it around her finger (making a doodle).

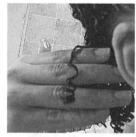

This is her adorable curl, nicely defined.

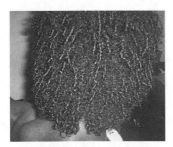

This is Frances before she puts doodles into her hair.

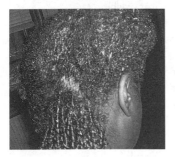

Frances has put conditioner in her hair and pinned up all of her hair except the section she's about to define.

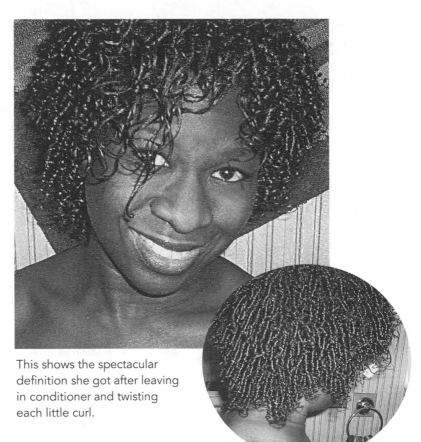

This shows the spectacular definition she got after leaving in conditioner and twisting each little curl.

long enough to form spirals and for very young children with short hair. I use this same technique on my shorter curls around the front of my face.

Shortcut, or for Looser Curls

If you have looser spirals (rather than tight circular coils), or if you just don't feel up to defining every curl individually, you can use a shortcut to styling your curls. Instead of smoothing each one, you can run your fingers through your hair to release the curls. Start with wet hair after you comb conditioner into it. Take a section of your hair, maybe a sixth of your hair or so, and run your fingers through your hair from scalp to ends, going section by section. You might want to run your fingers through it a

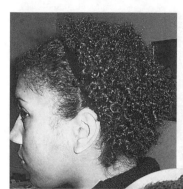

couple of times to divide your curls into smaller curl units. This helps separate your hair so that all of your curls won't be intertwined. They'll be free to do their own thing.

These photos are of the lovely Vanessa, a biracial woman living in Germany. Her hair is 100 percent natural, and she's never been to a hairdresser.

This photo was taken after Vanessa cut off her dreadlocks.

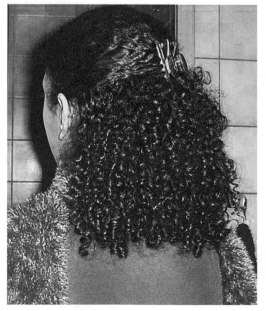

To set and define her curls after washing, applying conditioner, and combing, she says that she gently presses her fingers together as she runs her fingers through her hair. Pressing her fingers together actually helps form the curls when her hair slides through her fingers this way. She says, "When a section refuses to curl or looks fuzzy, I gently comb that section again so that it's really smooth, then rake [my fingers through] it once again."

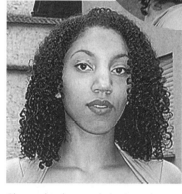

She styles her curls by running her fingers through them while wet, with conditioner in them. This is a perfect shortcut for people with curls loose enough to allow them to easily run their fingers through their wet hair.

Vanessa's hair from the back, as it's been growing out. It reaches to the middle of her back when she pulls it straight.

This is Dominique, who has loose curls. Curls like hers are perfect for just running your fingers through them a few times while they're wet with conditioner, to separate and define them. You can see that Dominique's curls are more defined and much calmer in the third picture. Dominique's mom, Amber, commented on using these techniques on her daughter's hair, saying, "Her curls are now soft, and all the curls are defined."

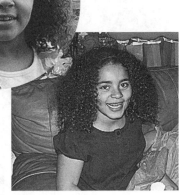

Dominique before her mom tried these techniques.

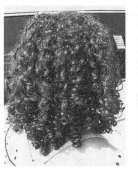

Dominique's defined curls from the back.

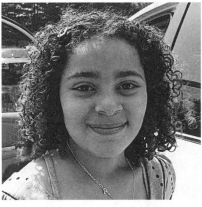

Dominique after her mom combed her hair with conditioner and left it in.

Good-bye to the Neon Part

All through grade school and high school, I had a big issue with parting my hair. You'd think something as simple as putting in a part would be no big deal. But while I was growing up, there was nothing easy about my hair, including parting it. Whenever I washed my hair, I had to figure out where to put my part while I was setting it with rollers. I had to decide right then where my part would go because once my hair was brushed into that chosen position, it was a battle to separate it into a new one.

After I had a part in a spot I liked, I tried really hard to keep it there. It wasn't easy to find a good spot for a part. It had to go at just the right

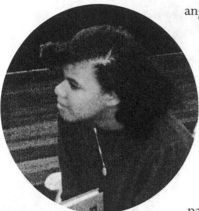

My fresh new part glows in my hair (about age fourteen).

angle, in exactly the right place. Because all of my hair was pressed down tightly on either side for control, the part looked huge. And when I did put in a new one, the new scalp that showed hadn't yet seen the sun (after being hidden beneath all of my hair). This meant that a new part was a disturbing neon-white color compared with my black hair and the rest of my tan skin. It looked like a fluorescent white stripe painted down the side of my head.

Now that I section my curls, there's no longer a part issue. My hair is now pre-sectioned into curls, and my part occurs wherever my hair happens to fall that day. And I can change it as often as I want. To go from a casual middle part (the way I usually wear my hair) to a side part, I just swing some curls over to the side. That's it. No more careful planning, doing several test runs, and then forcefully excavating a part for that week. Now my hair loosely parts right down the center on its own, whereas in the old relaxer days, my hair just seemed lost (and most likely terrified).

The Benefits of Defining with Conditioner

With your curls separated and reinforced, your hair can now move in the wind and shrug nonchalantly at drizzle. You can style it with ease and as an afterthought, instead of a battle. Each curl will be springy and smooth. Because your hairs aren't lots of loose and vulnerable individuals but are now curl units, they keep their shape. They can be pulled back into a bun or a braid (or several braids) at night while you sleep and still retain their shape in the morning when they're undone. (As a bonus, every day that you use conditioner to smooth and refresh your curls, your hair will be sweetly scented with the fragrance of your conditioner.) Heavy wind is not a disaster anymore. Instead of the wind whipping your hair into a frazzled cloud as it used to for me, it will merely toss each reinforced curl. At most, a little smoothing of your hairline with a bit of water and conditioner might be needed. Drizzle and even rain are no longer issues. Your hairs are locked together until they're combed again, and they're where they want to be. After being caught in the rain, you'll need to smooth your hair only to evenly distribute the moisture. But it's no big deal if you don't.

With your curls already defined, if there's a fuzzy spot or if a few curls get matted, it's easy to isolate the fuzzy parts. Then you can wet, recondition, and smooth them with your fingers or a comb. Previously, if I had a fuzzy spot, I'd have to tear it from the rest of my hair so that I could smooth it. That made a new problem: I'd snarled up all of the hair that I'd had to pull that section out of.

As you'll begin to realize when you start to smooth individual curls, leaving conditioner in your hair does four very important things: it makes your hair much easier to comb, it keeps your curls together without being crunchy or stiff, it conditions your hair, and it gives your curls weight.

- **Your hair is easier to comb (conditioner is slippery).** Conditioners are rich with emollients and filled with slippery ingredients. This is exactly what you need to get that comb to slide through your hair. Combing without conditioner is like running an engine's gears without oil. The strands of your hair need lubrication to help the teeth of your comb glide through them. It's also much easier to section your conditioned hair, because your curls slide apart more readily. Because your comb glides through your hair with less force, it means less stress is placed on your hair. Less stress means less damage.
- **Keeping curls together (so they don't puff apart) takes conditioner, not gel.** Conditioner works much better than gel for very curly hair. Conditioner keeps your curls smooth and clumped together but leaves them soft and conditioned. When you use gel to keep your curls together, the amount of product that's needed to achieve the same effect as conditioner would make your curls stiff and crunchy. And gels have very little conditioning ingredients, no matter what promises are written on the bottle.
- **Conditioner weighs down your hair.** Leaving conditioner in your hair gives your curls weight, so it gives a nice swing and

movement to spirals. If you want longer hair, it helps your coils flow down your back or sit on your shoulders. It does all of this without adding a greasy feel. It styles without feeling stiff and crunchy. As a bonus, your hair smells sweet, like your conditioner. Smoothing a little conditioner and water over your hair in the morning to refresh your curls and calm down fuzz makes your hair sleek and glossy and also refreshes the scent.

- **Conditioner is conditioning (your hair stays moisturized).** Combing conditioner through your hair means that every strand of your hair is coated with its moisturizing ingredients. Though your hair is very moisturized, however, it isn't greasy. That was a revelation to me. I'd always believed that moisturizing meant applying lots of hairdressing, and I had many oil-stained clothes and pillows to prove it. I cringed when someone wanted to touch my hair in the old days (which was rarely, mercifully), because I knew they'd be able to feel all of the oil I'd put on my hair to try to keep it from breaking off (which didn't work). Now, people come up to me all the time to feel my hair, and I'm more than happy to let them. (For more information about which conditioners are good for your hair and how to know which ingredients to look for, see chapter 11.)

- **Defining helps you monitor your ends.** By gliding your fingers over your curls to define them each week or so, it gives you a chance to check the condition of your ends. If a curl feels smooth all the way to the tip, you know you are treating your ends well, and they are sleek and happy. If you start to feel rough spots, it means either that you have a tangle within the curl that needs combing again or that damage may be occurring. Also, this is a great way to find all of those little hidden dot knots that can cluster on your ends. When I run across the tip of a curl that feels rough, it's often due to a cluster of these little knots (this happens to curly hair and doesn't mean you've done anything wrong unless all of your hair is covered in them). I snip off the end with the knots in it and keep going. Smoothing every week is your early warning system. It will let you know if and where a problem may be developing, and you will be able to catch it before much more damage occurs.

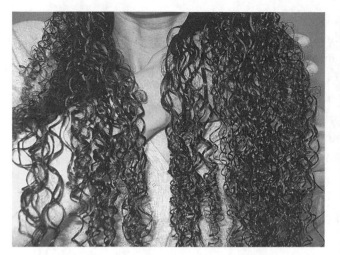

Done! After combing my hair, it looks a little stringy, and my curls are much looser than they would be if they were totally dry and I hadn't combed lots of conditioner into them. Remember, stringy is good. It means all of your curls are nicely set.

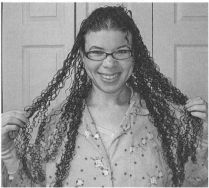

I also clip the front of my hair back (or wear a smooth plastic headband) to keep it from hanging in my face. If you want more height in the front, you can gently scrunch your curls forward (sort of pleating them in your hands) for lift before clipping them (with the scrunch still in them) off your face.

Troubleshooting the Puff

If your hair or any section of it is still puffing up (and you want a more defined look), here are a few tips to smooth out your curls:

- It does matter what kind of conditioner you use. Some can be too light, and others can get crunchy or sticky or build up in your hair. I've had the best results with the conditioners I recommend in chapter 11 or at TightlyCurly.com. If the conditioner is too light, it simply evaporates as if it was never there, instead of doing the job you need it to do.
- You might not be using enough conditioner. I really slather the conditioner into my sopping wet hair. (I don't even touch my hair with a towel; that's how wet my hair is when I comb it.) When you're combing in the conditioner, it will foam up if you're using enough of it to do the job. By the time you're done and you've finished defining and smoothing your curls, it vanishes. On the rare occasions when it doesn't, just dab a little water on those spots and wipe it away.

- If you're like me, you have a bunch of different-size curls all over your head. At the top and down the middle of my head, my curls are much smaller and tighter than anywhere else. These are the curls that are smaller than the diameter of a pencil. Because of this, when I separate my curls, I have to make the ones in this area much smaller than anywhere else. If I don't, they puff apart and then mat together. Sometimes I put as few as twenty strands of hair into each curl. Here's how I can tell the size of the curl I need to make: If I smooth a curl and it pops apart, then I know it's really two curls (or more) that I was trying to force into being one curl. I divide it again until each curl that I smooth stays together.
- Don't touch your curls while they dry; this is a crucial time when they're incubating.
- Make sure your hair dries completely before you put it up at night. This can take a while. I do my hair in the morning and go about my business the rest of the day. By the end of the day, my hair is dry.
- If your ends are puffing, you could smooth a little more conditioner back over them when they dry to reinforce their clumping. This often happens when the conditioner you're using to comb and set your hair with has a lighter, less emollient formula.
- If you've been wearing your hair in a style that's held it straight for some time, it may take your curls a few tries before they realize they've been set free. You might let some conditioner soak in them for an hour before you comb and define them. You could also scrunch them as you rinse in the shower and scrunch them even more as they dry. Hopefully, this will let them know they can curl back up again. It may take you a few attempts before your curls come back in full force.

Drying Your Curls

Once you have cleansed, conditioned, combed, and defined your curls, it's time to learn how to dry them and protect them. This insures that all of your careful work to define each gorgeous spiral will last throughout the week.

Air-Drying

The best way to dry your hair without damage is to let it dry naturally. Letting your hair air-dry keeps all of your strands still and calm, without the damaging temperatures and vigorous blowing from a hair dryer. The drawback to air-drying is that it can take four or more hours to do so, depending on the temperature and the humidity. I often comb my hair as early in the day as possible and then do my errands and chores while it dries.

If you want defined curls, leave your hair alone when it's drying! This is the time when your curls are vulnerable. Once they've set, they'll be strong and hold together, but until then, they're fragile. Not only should your hair never be combed during this time (or any time when it's dry), but don't even run your fingers through it. Do nothing that will separate your curls. Until your hair has dried—and preferably been slept on in buns or braids to give it a firm set—your hair is extremely vulnerable. The curls haven't set together yet, so if they get pulled apart and mussed, they'll stay separated and fuzzy and will probably mat in a few days.

Here are some tips to make the air-drying process successful. When your entire head of hair has been combed and separated, you can clip, or use a smooth headband, to keep the front hair back off your face if necessary. (I pin up the front of my hair to keep it out of my face, but also to add a little height at my crown.) Your hair will dry faster if it's kept loose so that air can get to all of your curls. If you'll be doing any physical activities, it's best to pull your hair back in a braid or a bun. When you're finished, you can take your hair back down again so that it can continue to dry.

It's best not to sleep on your hair when it's wet. I try to wash and comb my hair first thing in the morning so that I have the rest of the day for my hair to dry while I run errands. I've found that if I go to sleep with wet hair, I end up with a pancake head. Pressing down on my braided wet curls all night gives me a flat head. But even this is an improvement over the old days, when sleeping on my hair while it was wet meant that I'd have mats in the morning where my hair used to be.

Blow-Drying

You can occasionally blow-dry your hair, if necessary. Sometimes in the winter months, if it's very cold or damp and your hair is very thick, it might need a boost to fully dry. You can use a diffuser (these help keep curls in place) or a blow dryer set on low. When using the blow dryer, firmly hold the section of hair you're working on so that your curls don't whip around like they're in a tornado. It's best to concentrate on drying the hair at your scalp, because this hair is usually the last to dry. This gives your hair a jump-start on drying. Also, if the hair at your scalp is drier, it lifts all of the curls a bit. This is because dry hair expands a little, so more air can get in there to dry your hair.

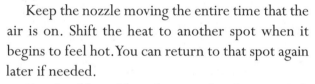

Hand Rule

To protect your hair when using heat, always follow the hand rule: if you blow the air on your hands, and it feels too hot there then it's most likely too hot to safely use on your hair.

Keep the nozzle moving the entire time that the air is on. Shift the heat to another spot when it begins to feel hot. You can return to that spot again later if needed.

You should not blow-dry your hair long enough for it to become absolutely dry. It's too easily damaged that way. I usually stop when my roots are barely damp instead of wet. Using a blow dryer in this way won't damage your hair as long as you're very careful. Remember, if the air feels too hot on your skin, it's too hot to be safe for your delicate hair.

Using a Diffuser

A diffuser is an excellent option for drying your curls. You can plop your hair down into the bowl of the diffuser and keep the setting on low. To protect your ends, you should concentrate on the hair at your scalp and leave your ends out to air-dry. Your ends will generally dry first anyway; it's the hair at the scalp that tends to need a little help sometimes.

With these cautions in mind, using a diffuser is a fine way to dry your hair sometimes. Just keep in mind that air-drying will never damage your hair, but anything that uses heat does have the potential to damage it.

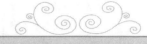

How to Keep Your Hair from Turning into a Mat When You Sleep

Curls snarl easily when left to their own devices. Curls especially don't like to get riled and knotted during the night. So, it's best to keep your hair smooth when you sleep to prevent matting. If you have very short hair that you want to grow out, you can sleep with it loose until it's long enough to pull back. Then you can smooth it and fasten it back with clips to keep it in place. Medium-length hair can be divided into two or more sections, then twisted into little buns or tiny braids. Longer hair can be pulled back into a firm braid if you're a restless sleeper or a simple bun or two fastened with a large tortoiseshell hairpin if you're a calm sleeper.

It's best to finish the ends of your night braids by twisting them together near the bottom. (Chapter 7 goes into more detail about creating a night braid to protect your ends and to keep them from snarling.)

Braid Bonus

A bonus to sleeping with your hair pinned smooth: if you want your curls to look longer, it "relaxes" them so that they'll hang a bit looser when you undo them in the morning.

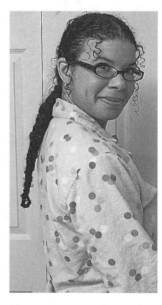

You can protect the ends of your braids by tucking them back into the lower braids in a loop to keep them safe from rubbing when you sleep.

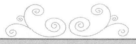

Braid Tips

Although it reduces tangles to put your hair back in a secure bun or braid when you sleep, never pull it so tightly back that you pull out all of your waves at the scalp by sheer force. You should never look like you're trying to give yourself a facelift from your hairstyle. This not only tortures your hair, akin to its being stretched out on a rack, but it also breaks your hair and will cause traction alopecia around your hairline. This means your hairline will get higher and higher as you lose more and more hair. By pulling your hair so tightly, you damage the roots to the point that they can't function any longer.

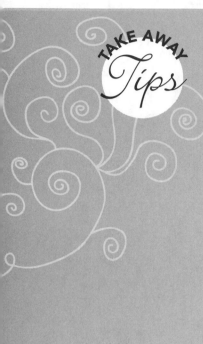

- Define your hair after you comb it with conditioner and while it is still very wet.

- Defining your curls reinforces their natural texture.

- Defining your curls helps you monitor them for damage.

- Conditioner weatherproofs your curls and gives them weight.

- Separating and defining your curls helps with styling (they're now pre-sectioned).

- Using conditioner to define curls saves money on gels, lotions, and mousses.

- For shorter hair, twist each section around your fingers (to make doodles).

- For a short cut, or for looser curls, you can run your fingers through your curls to define and separate them.

Chapter Seven

Everything Else
Daily Care and Beyond

For many of us, the relationship we have with our hair reaches deeper than simple adornment. Samson's hair held his strength, and Rapunzel engineered a rescue with hers. I equated having all of my hair cut off at age eleven to the end of my feral childhood, and the event served as an initiation into a deeply awkward adolescence.

Hairstyles across cultures might symbolize familial ties, tribal identity, marital status, social status, and even political beliefs. People of many cultures braid or twist amber, silver coins, and colorful glass beads into their hair, so hair styles are an art form, as well as a display of status and wealth. Our hair conveys our personalities on a more profound level than our clothes can. Although an outfit might express our mood on the day we wear it, our hair, by its continual presence, becomes an extension of ourselves. Our hair speaks of us in a silent complex of signifiers based on how we choose to display it. Danièle Pomey-Rey describes hair in *The Science of Hair Care* as being "midway between nature and culture, between skin and clothing." Our hair feels as if it has its own personality. A crown of thriving curls seems to radiate energy and vitality.

Because the way we wear our hair expresses our personalities to those around us, it makes sense to display it in the most flattering ways possible. Mangled hair that looks as if it's barely tolerated by its owner will communicate differently from the way radiant curls that appear loved and full of joy will. Learning how to let our curls sing instead of stifling them happens only when we take the time to listen to what they need—and act on it. The tips in this chapter can make it easier for you to style your curls from day to day, and I've also thrown in a few fun ideas.

Everyday Care

Once your hair is cleansed, conditioned, combed, defined, and dried, the daily upkeep is minimal. Since you've given your curls the go-ahead to do what they wanted to do all along, they will stay curled and clumped together. Now that your curls are doing what they were born to do, you don't need to do much daily upkeep. Following are a few tips to help you and your curls enjoy each other during the week.

Braiding Tips

To keep your hair from matting up at night while you sleep, it needs to be protected by putting it in several buns if it's shorter or one bun if it's longer. If you're a restless sleeper, a big braid or two is more secure. Putting your hair into either buns or braids at night is also a great way to help relax your curls if you want your hair to hang longer. Because the ends of your hair are snarl-prone, you can finish off the last couple of inches in a twist: braid your hair all the way down to the last two inches from the end. Then take the three sections of the braid and combine the two smallest sections together. As you do so, give the combined segments a twist to help meld them into one piece. Then wrap them around each other in a two-strand twist down to the end. To protect these fragile ends from rubbing against your pillow, you can loop them up and tuck them back into the braid (you can see how I do my night braid, below).

I have reached the last couple of inches of my hair. I now want to turn the braid into a twist, to make it easier to take out later.

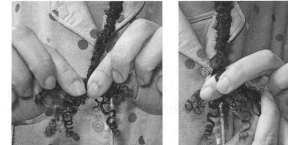

I combine the two smallest sections into one and give them a little twist together before I continue.

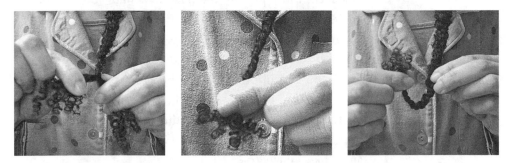

I continue to twist the two remaining sections down to the ends.

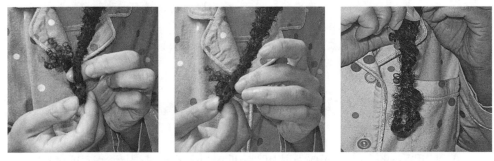

When you reach the ends of your curls, loop up the ends and tuck them into your braid. (I don't twist down to the very tips, because they will tangle too easily.) This will protect your fragile ends from rubbing against the sheets.

Unbraiding the Tips

When you unbraid your hair in the morning, keep in mind that this activity involves the ends, a notorious tangling zone. All of your tightest spirals will most likely be here, waiting to wrap themselves inextricably together. To prevent this from happening, here are a couple tips for undoing your night braid in the morning.

First, it's best to take a nickel-size dollop of conditioner, add a little water to it, and smooth this over the ends of your braid. Spirals are at their tightest when completely dry. This step will keep the ends slippery and a bit looser to prep your ends for being undone. Think of it as almost like giving them a little sleeping pill before you load them into their carrier for the trip to the vet.

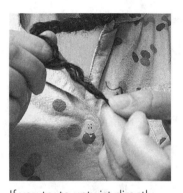

If you try to untwist directly from the top down without holding your ends in place, they'll snarl with ferocity. By controlling the ends as you open your twist, they don't get a chance to whirl around one another and knot into a rosette.

Left on their own, your curl ends get confused and will grab at one another in a panic. With your soothing guidance, you'll prevent them from tangling. Before you begin to unbraid, hold the very tip of your braid. Open up the twist near where it meets the braid, then gently run your finger down to the end. Continue to hold the braid's tip in your other hand. When you've untwisted as far as you can, it's now safe to let the tip finish untwisting the rest of the way in your other hand. Open up your fingers a little to let the tip untwirl under your guidance, like a curly top.

If your ends tend to be very tangly, instead of releasing them to let them twirl open in your fingers, you can untwist them manually. Turn them with your fingers in the direction they want to untwist.

Morning Hair

Morning used to be a stressful time for me back when I was using chemicals. It once seemed that no matter how I set my hair at night, come morning, it was stiff and I couldn't find a way to style it. The ends fanned open at broken angles, and every day was a challenge to find a way to hide as much of my hair (especially those fractured ends) as possible. Now that my hair is natural, it takes me only a few seconds to do my hair, and I don't have to give it much thought at all. I make sure my coiled ends show every day, because I'm so happy to have them. It amazes me what a difference learning to love my hair for what it is has made in my life.

Refresh Your Morning Curls

The last step to having easy to care for hair that lasts all week is to refresh your curls every morning. Once your hair is unbraided, it's time to prepare your curls for the day. You don't need to rinse your hair, or recomb it. If your hair looks fuzzy, you'll simply smooth over it with water and conditioner. To smooth it, take about a quarter-size squirt of conditioner in the palm of your hand and add some water. Rub your hands together and smooth the watery conditioner over your hair. You might find that you need to concentrate on the top part of your hair, closest to your scalp, because that's what usually gets the fuzziest. Then go back, get a little more watery conditioner, and smooth it over your ends.

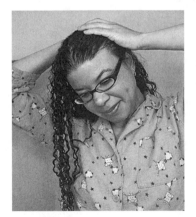

First, I wet my hands and smooth over the front of my hair. Then I do the same with a little conditioner.

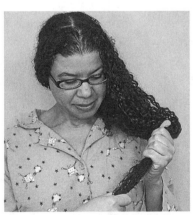

Next, I wet my hands and smooth over my ends, then follow with conditioner. You can vary the amount of water and conditioner, depending on what's needed.

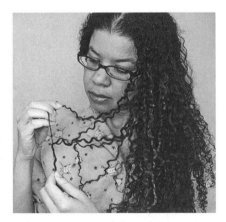

If you need to separate any of your curls, make sure to hold the bottom of both curls, and gently pull one curl away from the other.

If some ends have gotten mashed or fuzzy, concentrate on smoothing water and conditioner over the fuzziest parts. You can gently finger-comb the wet, conditioned ends if any of them have snarled. If your ends are really tangled, apply a bit more conditioner and water, and either work through the troubled curls with your fingers or gently comb out only those tangled ends. Concentrate on the tangled ends. This returns them to their original coils. When you unbraid your hair in the morning, it might look as if all of your curls are unfocused or have melded into part of the braid pattern and the half-curl pattern. This is only temporary. Once you smooth a little water and conditioner over them, they'll curl right back up as if they had never been braided overnight, except that they will hang a little longer overall.

You can smooth your hair with conditioner first, then go back over it again with water or with water and then conditioner. It's no big deal if you put in too much conditioner; simply smooth more water over it afterward. This spreads the conditioner throughout your hair. A big bonus is that you get to start your day smelling like your favorite conditioner.

When you put your hair up at night in a bun or a braid, I like to think that it goes to sleep when you do. When you undo your braid or bun in the morning, all of your little curls are still sleeping, so they'll look sort of flattened. When you smooth over your hair with water and conditioner, your curls wake up. By the time your hair dries, your curls will have returned to their coily selves. I've found that the more water I smooth on them, the tighter they curl back up, and the more conditioner I smooth over them, the more defined the ends become. Drenching the ends of your hair every day so that they are dripping wet, however, will dry them out over time. This step covers your basic hair-care routine, and it should last you all week when you refresh your pretty curls every morning.

The Overhang

If your hair tends to hang in your face like a mud flap when you wear it down, as mine does, regular gels might be too wimpy to keep it in place. Use a dime-size glop of spiking putty, and smooth it in at your front hairline—where all of that holding action needs to take place. Lightly run your fingers over the hair of your hairline, and even poke your fingers into your hairline (only) as you apply the putty. Put three or four clips here while it dries. You can push your hair forward to emphasize the curls at your hairline, giving them a nice lift before you clip them into place. When your hair is dry and set, take the clips out. This is important: No combing or finger-combing while it dries or after it's dry!

I try to style my hair off my face only on very rare occasions. It usually takes longer than the one minute or so per day I spend on my hair the rest of the week. On the few times when I've tried this, my hair usually ended up flopping into my face by the end of the day anyway. I tend to go for the easiest styles for me to do, so I normally just let my hair part down the middle and I let it be (see "Basic Loose Style" in chapter 13).

Deep Conditioning

I know it feels as if your hair is alive, with a personality all its own. Technically, though, your hair isn't alive, so it can't repair itself. No magic product can repair your hair once it's been hurt. Your hair is like a fabric made of keratin. Hoping that you can repair damaged hair with magical products is as realistic as soaking a torn sweater in yarn and expecting it to mend. Luckily for us, hair continues to grow. So even though you'll never be able to grow a new sweater in your closet, you'll eventually get a new head of hair.

It turns out that nearly all of the ingredients that are in deep conditioners are often the very same ingredients that are in that brand's regular conditioner. It's just that they often package it differently and charge more for it.

Once you stop damaging your hair, deep conditioning isn't necessary. If you feel like giving your hair a treat sometimes, though, your hair won't mind a bit. Deep conditioning can be simple or elaborate. You can apply a very easy oil treatment by using natural massage oils you might have lying around the house, cooking oils, or commercially available hot oil treatments for hair. Smooth any of these oils over your hair, concentrating on the ends. Then step into the shower and wash it out.

For more conditioning, pin up your hair and let the oil sit in it for as long as you like. Do some chores or take it easy and watch television before you wash the oil out. For an even deeper treatment, place a plastic bag or a shower cap over your hair to seal in body heat, or even wrap a hot towel, with the water wrung out of it, over your head. This can be done for a few minutes or hours before you wash your hair. (You might need to apply a little more shampoo than usual when it's time to wash the oil out.) Follow the oil treatment with conditioning and continue to do your hair as usual.

Another good and very simple way to condition your hair is to put about one-half teaspoon of natural oil into a full bottle of the conditioner you're using. Shake it vigorously to mix it. Most of the time, though, I don't get around to putting oil in any of my conditioners. Contrary to what I was taught, heavy grease and oils (such as petroleum, shea butter, lanolin, plant oils, or heavy silicones) can build up when you put them thickly on your scalp, and if they don't get washed off thoroughly, they can clog your hair follicles, actually damaging the growth of your hair.

What I do to add a bit more conditioning, especially in the winter, is put a little olive oil on my ends before braiding my hair up at night. Another excellent oil to use is coconut oil, which studies have shown penetrates the hair shaft to help strengthen it.

It's funny now, because during my adolescence, I used hairdressing products fanatically. I firmly believed that if I could find the right brand, my hair would finally grow. (Well, all the jars of product kept telling me so.) Every night I'd divide my hair into sections, work finger-scoops of the dressing into every section, and then set my hair. My chemically treated hair used to feel like crunchy threads without the hairdressing products. With them, my hair felt like oiled crunchy threads.

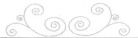

Money-Saving Tip

Occasionally adding a little oil to your routine is a good way to use up recently expired olive oil or other exotic cooking oils such as walnut oil, or massage oil that isn't being otherwise used. Be careful not to put in too much, or your hair might end up feeling oily.

My hair reaches past my tailbone today, and I didn't use hairdressing products to grow it to this length. In fact, I haven't used any of these products since I cut off my chemically damaged hair more than ten years ago. I use conditioner alone, and now my hair shines all the way to the ends. Leaving in the conditioner eliminates the need to use hairdressing.

Scalp Issues

If you have scalp problems, I suggest that you first see a dermatologist. My hair-care tips are in no way a substitute for heeding a doctor's advice. If you have a flaky scalp, however, you can try using a dandruff shampoo instead of regular shampoo. Because, with these techniques, you're shampooing only your scalp anyway (and chasing that with a conditioner rinse), medicated shampoo won't dry out the rest of your hair. Even so, try to get a conditioning type of dandruff shampoo if possible. And again, make certain to apply the medicated shampoo only to your scalp, because these types of products can be extremely drying.

Shampoo without Shampooing

If you're washing your hair about once or twice a week with a medicated shampoo and you continue to have flaking, there's a way you can cheat a little. You can apply medicated shampoos more frequently without having to wash and comb all of your hair each time. The secret is that you don't have to wash your hair every time you wash your scalp. You can wash only the front and the sides of your hairline, which frees you to do it more often, if necessary. This is best to do in the morning, when you'll most likely be wetting your hair to smooth it back anyway.

Start by pulling your hair back in a firm bun, or clip it back if it's shorter, so that your hair is secure and far away from your face. Wet the front of your scalp, areas around your hairline, and the sides—any place you can easily get to and can fit under the faucet of the sink. Apply your medicated shampoo, always with gentle fingers, and work it under the hair of your hairline as much as possible. Scrub gently, working the lather into the scalp. If there's time, you could let it sit for a few minutes (make sure the directions say that's okay). Then put your head under the faucet, and rinse the sudsy areas very carefully. Be careful not to get too enthusiastic and wet the rest of your hair. Afterward, smooth conditioner over your hair to slick it down and moisturize it again.

You can also do this at night, but then you might end up with a damp pillow. Follow the previous directions, and afterward towel-blot your hair to remove most of the water. Smooth a little conditioner over the washed areas to keep them moist. If your hair is too short to pull back to ensure that it doesn't mat, slick it back with clips. In the morning, smooth water over it with a little more conditioner for any fuzzing that popped up overnight.

To make things easier on yourself, you could keep one type of dandruff shampoo by your sink to use every day or every other day in the mornings. One bottle could have one type of active ingredient in it, and the other one, another active ingredient. Always test them to make sure you don't have any allergic reactions to either or both products combined. This technique is especially useful if you tend to put lots of heavy products directly and generously on your scalp (see "Deep Conditioning," above). Washing the hair-conditioning products off every few days will keep them from building up and clogging the pores of your scalp (which could potentially stunt your hair's growth).

Occasional Care: Trimming

The purpose of trimming hair is to get rid of damaged ends. Using the techniques in this book will eliminate any damage being done to your hair. Therefore, if you follow these techniques, you won't need to trim your hair—that is, if your goal is to grow your hair long. The exception is if you still have damaged hair remaining from previous styling techniques. Then the damaged hair will need to be removed. Once your hair is healthy, however, you won't need to trim it unless you want to maintain a particular shorter length.

Here's why: Hair grows about one-half inch a month. People are often told they should trim their ends one-half inch every month or two. In this case, your hair would be trimmed off nearly as fast as it grows in. This is absolutely necessary if you're gradually cutting off your damaged and/or permed hair, especially if you don't feel comfortable cutting it off all at once. If you have strong, undamaged, virgin growth, however, trimming isn't necessary. If your hair isn't being damaged, then the trim would merely remove perfectly good hair.

On top of that, if you go to a salon to get your hair trimmed, you most likely will encounter someone who is unfamiliar with very curly hair or impatient about the time it takes to comb curls. This person might be tempted to rapidly rip a comb through your hair, which would do more damage to your hair than would leaving your ends in their current state. Besides, curls are self-replacing. The life span of a strand of hair is about six or seven years, on average. This means that about every six years, you have a totally new head of hair from the one you had six years ago, depending on the life span of your hair. So even if there's a little damage, in a few years that hair will be replaced by new growth anyway. And remember, the techniques in this book give you damage-free hair. The purpose of trimming is to cut off the damaged ends. If there's no damage, trimming isn't necessary.

Curls are forgiving, so trimming can cut away a lot of length unnecessarily. For straight hair, keeping it cut and trimmed *is* important, because split and uneven ends show up easily; the hair is uniform and all in a row. Little can be hidden with straight hair. Curls are vastly more forgiving. Sections with a tighter curl will look shorter than sections with a looser curl. Each curl will curl in its own unique way, hundreds of times over your head, so there's no way to spot minor unevenness.

If you're trying to grow your hair long, there's also the sacrifice of length to consider. If, without trimming, hair grows one-half inch a month, with a life span of about six years per strand, provided it isn't damaged, your hair has the potential to grow about thirty-six inches, or three feet long. If you trimmed your hair regularly one-half inch every other month for those six years, it would cut away nearly eighteen inches, or about one and one-half feet, of hair. That's nearly half of all the new growth you'd produce during that time.

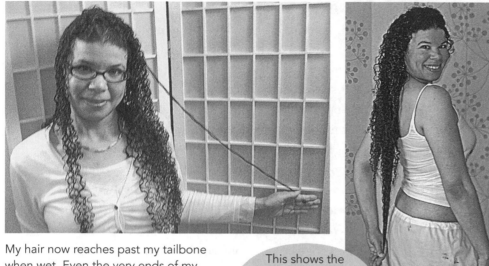

My hair now reaches past my tailbone when wet. Even the very ends of my coils shine. I haven't trimmed my hair in more than ten years.

This shows the length of my hair. When wet, it's down to my thighs.

Damaged hair—and hair that continues to be damaged—will always need trimming, however. As long as depilatory-strength chemicals have been eating away at a head of hair, trimming will need to be done. When you eliminate damage, there's no longer a need to trim. This means that when you do eliminate the damage, in time your hair could grow long enough to sit on.

Commando Hair Care: Trimming It Yourself

Depending on how curly your hair is, you may be able to cut it yourself, as long as you will always wear it curly (curls are forgiving—straight hair isn't). I used to trim my hair myself back in the days when I was trimming it. I also sometimes asked a friend with straight hair to do the trimming for me, using the following method. Try this only if your hair is very curly, however, and if you don't plan to wear it straight. You should err on the side of cutting much less than you planned to until you get the hang of estimating how much your hair draws up when dry.

What You Will Need

- A spray bottle with water in it
- Conditioner
- Good, sharp hair-cutting scissors
- Clips to pin hair back
- A ruler (optional)
- A towel to go over your shoulders and to catch snips.

How to Trim It Yourself

- Make sure your hair is wet and combed with conditioner in it (trimming is great to do after washing and combing your hair with conditioner).
- Pick up each curl and hold it firmly between your fingers, stretching it open.
- Position your scissors so that the blades will be straight across all of the hairs.
- Give each curl a snip, so that the scissors cut straight across your hairs in a "T" shape.
- Take off much less than you think you should, because curls shrink up to a fraction of their wet length when dry. It's impressive how much they shrink, so be very careful.
- Lift up the curls on either side of your head from time to time to make sure both sides are even.
- Pin back the snipped curls so that they don't get re-snipped.
- Work your way through your whole head until all of the ends have been snipped.
- Check frequently to make sure both sides are even.
- You can use the ruler to make sure both sides of your hair are even.

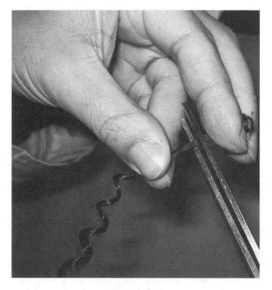

Hold your curl open and make a "T" shape when cutting between your hair and the scissors.

Framing Your Face

When your hair gets longer, you might want to have a few wispy curls to frame your face. These curls are fun. Because they're short, and you don't intend to grow them long like the rest of your hair, you don't have to be as careful with them as with the rest of your curls. They can stay out when you sleep and when you shower. They'll pop out randomly when your hair is pulled back, giving a softer, more romantic look to your hairstyles, and they are a great way to showcase how adorable your coils are.

The best way to cut your curls is with restraint first, scissors second. Start with only the tiniest amount of hair for your bangs; otherwise, they have the potential to get big and fuzzy and hard to manage.

With your hair down, take the end of a tortoiseshell hairpin, a comb, a knitting needle, or anything else with a thin but rounded point that can divide hair without stabbing you. Part your front hair into the very thinnest continuous line of hair possible. Start from your middle part all the way to your ears—if you want wisps to frame your face. If you want only bangs, separate out the thinnest continuous line of hair from across your forehead. When you've separated one side of your wisps-to-be from the rest of your hair, pin up your hair, leaving out your separated hair. Do the same to the other side of your hair.

Where you choose to cut depends on how curly your hair is. If your curls are tight, keep your sections longer than if your hair tends to be wavy around your hairline. It's better to err on the long side. If the curls are not short enough, you can always go back and snip off a little more.

You'll do one-half of your hair and then the other, using the first half as a template to cut the other.

The best place to start cutting is at the hair that falls from directly above your eyes. Pull the hair that grows

These two curls grow side by side, and they are both cut to chin length. You can see how the curlier one draws up tighter than the looser curl does. Keep this in mind when you're cutting your hair.

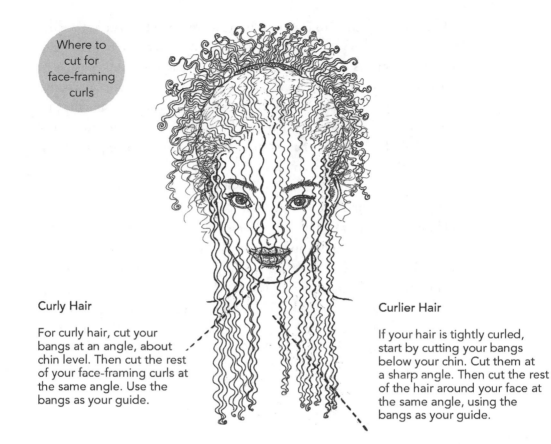

Where to cut for face-framing curls

Curly Hair

For curly hair, cut your bangs at an angle, about chin level. Then cut the rest of your face-framing curls at the same angle. Use the bangs as your guide.

Curlier Hair

If your hair is tightly curled, start by cutting your bangs below your chin. Cut them at a sharp angle. Then cut the rest of the hair around your face at the same angle, using the bangs as your guide.

from your forehead down to your chin in one hand. It's best to leave some slack in your hair when you hold it. This way, if it turns out a bit too long, you can trim a little more. If your hair tends to coil up tightly like a seashell when it's shorter than a certain length, and you cut your hair shorter than that length, you'll have little curl-shells along your hairline instead of wisps, and you won't be able to put any back. Leaving in some slack ensures that there's still extra length built into the cut as a precaution against this happening.

Take your scissors and cut at an angle. Start from your chin (if your curl is looser) or below your chin (if it's curlier) and head downward, at a slope. The shortest part should be the hair that grows closest to your center part. Your hair should get longer as you approach the hair that grows from the area above your ears.

Use this cut section to line up your next cut. Take the hair at the edge of the cut (closer to your ears than to your center part) and hold it beside the hair that grows from your temples. Cut this at the same angle, with your hair being left longer as you approach your ears. Take the section between your temple and ears and cut this hair at an angle, using the previous section as your guide. Use this half to measure where to cut the rest of your hair. Because your hair is curly, it doesn't have to be perfect; the curls will all curl different amounts anyway.

When you wash and comb your hair, it's okay to comb your bangs into the rest of your hair. Different pieces will randomly fall from your hair and will look more natural this way. If, after a week, no wisps have popped out of place, you might want to go back and cut a thicker line of hair this time. You could even select a few wispy pieces when you comb your hair and separate these from the other curls.

I cut my wispy hairs myself. They aren't perfect, but it doesn't matter. I enjoy having them. Some sections are really curly, and then a section right next to those might be merely wavy. Different curls come out every time I comb my hair.

Swimming

It isn't so much the swimming that's hard on your hair, but what's in the water and how you handle your hair afterward. Saltwater is corrosive if left on your hair too long (think of what happens to cars driven on salt-covered snowy roads). Chlorine is also damaging. After you swim in water that contains salt or chlorine, the main objective is to get those substances out of your hair as soon as possible. The second major concern is tangling.

What You Will Need to Care for Your Hair after Swimming

- An oil such as olive, coconut, jojoba, a natural massage oil, or a type of silicone (for example, dimethicone)
- A hair clip to hold the ends of your hair in place
- Shampoo (clarifying or swimmer's shampoo is good but not necessary)

- Lots of light conditioner
- Lots of heavy conditioner
- A Denman-type brush

The best way to wear your hair while you swim is to coat it lightly with an oil such as coconut, olive, jojoba, a natural massage oil, or a silicone like dimethicone, which puts a protective coating on your hair (these oils don't rinse off easily in water, so they stay put even in water to protect it). Then put it in one or two firm braids. Don't pull your hair tight, just firm enough so that your hair won't unravel in the water and get really tangled. Then braid your hair gently all the way to the ends to hold it in place.

When you are finished swimming, wash your scalp with shampoo as usual. (The exception to the shampooing is if you swam in freshwater and it isn't time to wash your hair yet. You can skip shampooing and simply do a good wash using conditioner instead of shampoo.) When your hair and scalp are rinsed thoroughly, wash your hair several times with the light conditioner, making sure to squeeze it into your hair. Rinse, then follow with your heavy-duty conditioner. Leave this in and comb and define your curls as usual.

Camping

Camping often involves being away from showers or even a steady source of water, and most likely there isn't time or room to carry the needed supplies to comb out your hair. Also, if you have a child going to summer camp for a few weeks, she might not yet be able to comb and define her curls on her own or even have the opportunity. The best thing to do when out in the middle of the woods is to keep your hair as calm and contained as possible.

Minimal Hair Items for Camping (if you won't have time to comb)
- A small bottle (about 1 ounce or so) of combing conditioner
- A tiny bottle of a natural oil such as coconut or olive oil

Before going on your trip, wash and comb your hair with a good conditioner, and let your hair dry completely. Because your hair will most likely be up for the entire trip, you can simply finger-define your curls to save time. It's important to let it totally dry—it will be braided for a while, and it wouldn't be good for it to go sour because it was put up wet. After your hair totally dries, put it in a night braid (see "Braiding Tips" in this chapter). If you won't have the resources to wash and comb your hair, then don't take your hair out of this braid. The more you can keep your hair still, the less matted it will get, even if you are away for a couple weeks (if you are away for longer than this, you might want to bring your combing supplies).

On the morning of your trip, don't take out your braid. Just undo a few inches of hair at the bottom of your braid and smooth with a little water and combing conditioner. Then, every night, braid your ends back up and tuck them into the rest of your braid to protect them. If you are in a dry climate, smooth a little coconut or olive oil on the ends before braiding. In the morning, you can undo a few inches of the ends and smooth them with a little water and conditioner to refresh your curls. At the end of the week, simply unbraid, then rebraid your hair to keep it looking smooth.

Tips before Going to a Salon

I know I'm paranoid, but I don't go to salons anymore. I don't see the point in it. I've learned to take care of my hair without damaging it, and my hair thrives. All of my experiences in salons damaged my hair or my dignity or both, and the information I was given was often alarmingly wrong. The standard techniques used by salons seem to be one method fits all. Unfortunately, our hair isn't like everyone else's hair. With the techniques in this book, you won't need to go to salons anymore, and you'll save lots of money doing your hair yourself. If you need to get your hair cut, though, I'll give you some tips and ideas.

The biggest problem we have when we go to salons is that our curly hair is difficult to comb. Some hairdressers have never worked with hair like ours before, so they don't know that little combs simply won't go through our hair without causing us severe pain and damaging our hair.

A "regular" hairdresser might not be trained in how to handle very curly hair, because it generally isn't included in stylists' training. They might even try to comb your hair with a fine-toothed comb or start combing at the top of your hair. My best advice is, if a stylist tries to do this to your hair, power walk yourself out of there, knowing that she has no idea about your curls and will end up hurting you, your hair, and her comb.

If you do visit a salon, however, here are some lessons I've learned that might help you through the experience.

Questions and Research

Before going to a salon, you *could* ask whether its hairdressers handle very curly hair, but in my experience, they all say yes. Even stylists who have no idea what to do with our hair say they do. Stylists whose only experience with our hair consists of once having seen a photo in a magazine of someone with hair like ours, years ago, will still say yes. It's frustrating, but I've found this to be true. Mildly curly hair is often called extremely curly, because people have no other reference point. So, when you ask stylists whether they've worked on extremely curly hair, they feel that they have. I've never had stylists tell me they *weren't* familiar with curls like mine, even when I found out later that they had no idea what to do with them. I've heard stories of biracial women going to salons with well-known curl-expert stylists, and the stylists ended up getting overwhelmed and frustrated by the amount of volume contained in very curly hair. The customers walked out with their feelings hurt.

One way to find a salon that works with your kind of hair is to ask someone with very curly hair where she gets her hair done—if you can find anyone. The reality is that you might be the only person who looks like you in your area. I have yet to find someone in Seattle with hair like mine. I also didn't see anyone with hair like mine in Sacramento or Santa Cruz. I'm sure they were there, but I simply never saw them. Instead of merely asking stylists whether they've worked with curly hair, it might be best to question them on *how* they approach curly hair:

- Do they start combing from the top or the bottom?
- What sort of comb do they use: fine-toothed or one with wide teeth?

- Are they patient? If you don't want to ask this outright (especially since they'll most likely answer yes, no matter how impatient they really are), ask them how long they usually spend combing curly hair. Sometimes salons that spend more time cost more, but I believe they're worth it. (Be sure to tip well if your stylist takes her time with your hair, because this person is a treasure!)
- Ask whether they cut curly hair wet or flat-iron it dry before cutting. (Make sure they don't flat-iron wet hair, because it can boil the water in your hair and produce tiny bubbles that will cause your hair to break off (see chapter 2).

Pre-Combing

As mentioned, some salons might straighten your hair with a hot comb or blow it dry before cutting it. I feel these are highly damaging, so I'd to go to a place that cut my hair wet (if, that is, I went anywhere). Right before going, you will probably want to comb your hair first, with conditioner, and keep it wet. Then, when you go into the salon, it won't take nearly as long for the stylist to get a comb through your locks. Make sure your hair stays wet. If your hair is short or less curly, you should be able to skip this step, because it doesn't take nearly as long to comb short curly hair or looser curls as it does long or tightly curly hair.

Beware!

Under no circumstances should you let yourself get talked into having a chemical applied to your hair to straighten it. Astoundingly, hairstylists are often uninformed about how the chemicals work and what they do, so they'll tell you the wrong thing. Sometimes (and I know this is my paranoia talking) I feel as if hairdressers are on a mission to wipe out all curls from the planet, and to them the only acceptable way for hair to be is straight, by any means necessary. I've been told twice, in different states and at different times, that applying a relaxer to my hair would keep my curls exactly as they are and would only make it easier to run a comb through them. And the relaxer wouldn't damage my hair; the stylists promised this emphatically.

And at these times—one time, I already had a texturizer in my hair, and another time I was trying to grow out my hair in high school—I wanted so much for this to be true that I let them put the chemicals in my hair. All it did was help ruin my hair.

A relaxer, a straightener, a texturizer, or a kiddie perm takes the curls out of your hair and in return leaves it damaged. Anything that permanently changes your hair damages it. It's that simple. When your hair is damaged, it's harder to comb and far more fragile. You might not see the damage immediately and might walk out of the salon with bouncing, swinging, wavy hair. But in a few months the cancer will have had time to do its work. Your hair will become shorter and duller, and when you comb, it will feel as if there's a thin coating of grit on your hair. So, don't let stylists mislead you. Be paranoid—like me.

Watch the Scissors

It's best to keep your eagle eyes on how much of your hair is being cut. This is no time to be passive. It's your hair. Fight for it! Keep your eye on the length of hair that falls on your shoulders when it's being trimmed. Don't wait until *after* the stylist spins you around to face the mirror to discover that you both misunderstood how much length was to be removed.

Curly wet hair hangs much longer than curly dry hair does. Stylists who are unfamiliar with how much your hair coils back up when it's dry may cut your wet hair thinking that the way it looks while wet is similar to where it will end up when dry. This is often not the case. Know how much your hair draws up when drying. Again, keep eagle eyes on those scissors.

The Layering Question

Many times, well-meaning people suggest layering our hair to help manage it. This is a myth. There is no magic cut, no product, no tool that will suddenly enable us to treat our hair as straight-haired people treat theirs.

There just isn't. Our hair is curly, and we have to treat it like curly hair. People often say that layering will help "release the curls" in your hair, meaning that when you comb it all together, because different sections are of different lengths, those curls will be forced to curl separately from one another. What will most likely happen, with your tight curls, is that you will get several levels of hair, resembling stair steps on your head. This is because each section was cut differently, so it will have a different length of curl. The less length (weight), the tighter the curl. Therefore, the shortest layers will be drawn up tightly, like a fist on the back of your head. The next-shortest layer will be drawn up slightly less and will curl at a slightly different level. The next-longest layer will curl at another degree of tightness. Depending on the tightness of your curl, the differences in the levels that are now cut into your hair could be drastically pronounced. And the shortest layers will have the tightest curls, making that layer look even shorter and puffier. The longest layer will have the loosest curls, making it look even longer. If you have very loose curls, layers might work fine for you. Or, at the most, you could have them cut off in very small amounts per layer, with maybe only an inch difference between them to be safe. But I strongly caution those of us with tighter coils against it.

The main point is, because you've now learned to manually separate all of your curls, you don't have to wait for a "cure-all" haircut to separate them for you. Because your curls are unique, the best styles are those that show them off, not ones that layer them.

Long Hair Care

It was an amazing moment when I felt the weight of my hair resting between my shoulder blades for the first time. Along with the excitement, however, comes additional mindfulness. The ends are the oldest part of your hair and need as much protection as possible. Curly long hair must be watched as you would a curious toddler. Long curls will pull objects off tables, catch in branches as you pass them, and wrap around your buttons as you put on a shirt. Long curls will tangle in your clothes as you are dressing or get caught in your bra as you put it on. Being longer means each curl has a longer reach with which to grab and catch onto things. When your hair gets long enough, it can give you a big shock, as it did to me: a few months ago, while I was washing it in the shower, my wet hair swung back and slapped me on my behind.

In addition to your hair's potential for mischief, you must be more aware of keeping the ends from harm. Long hair can get damaged in many ways you wouldn't think of. A few damaging situations to protect your hair from include catching it

- Between your back and the seat of a chair.
- Between your chest and your arms when you cross your arms.
- When someone puts his or her arm around your shoulders.
- Under the strap of an over-the-shoulder bag, purse, or luggage.
- In a car door when you close it.
- In your clothes, bra, buttons, hooks, or zipper. (When you're dressing or trying on clothes, it's best to put your hair up in a quick bun to get it out of harm's way.)
- Inside the sleeves of coats and sweaters.
- In a seatbelt when you buckle it.

You never know; you might inspire other tightly curled people to embrace their curls. Maybe seeing how proudly you wear your curls and how beautiful they are might provide someone with the needed incentive to give her own curls a try. How I wish I'd known a woman with curls like mine when I was a child! I wish I could have seen what they *could* have been—if only I'd known what to do. It would have given me such hope. Instead, I spent most of my life ashamed of my curls and feeling punished by them. If only I'd known how wonderful they were! If only I'd known that my hair is unique, not an aberration. You could be that inspiration to a child or a young person who's looking for a positive affirmation for a feature that has made her feel singled out her entire life. Because of you, someone could learn what a beautiful gift her curls really are.

- Put your hair up in buns or braids when you sleep.

- To undo your braid, use conditioner and water, and gently guide open your ends.

- To perk up your curls in the morning, smooth them with conditioner and water.

- You don't need to trim your hair if you stop damaging it.

- Stylists will tell you they can do your hair, even when they can't.

- Research before you put your hair in anyone's hands. Watch, ask questions, be paranoid, and be prepared to run.

Chapter Eight

Baby Curls
Tips for Little Ones

'm so glad you're reading this! Take it from a once-curly kid (now a curly adult), the best thing you can do for a child with tightly curly hair is to help her learn to care for her own natural curls. You will be giving her much more than healthy hair in the process.

Caring for tightly curly hair is not the same as caring for straight or wavy hair. This means that hair care for a child with tight curls will take a little more time. Yet once you know what curls need, understanding how to properly care for them is no longer a mystery. Soon your little one will have ringlets and coils spilling down her back, and other parents will be coming up to you to ask how you did it.

Showing a very curly child how to best take care of her curls is essential in helping her feel comfortable in her own body. It isn't enough to simply tell a child she is beautiful, yet treat her as if the hair (or any other part of her, for that matter) that she was born with is unacceptable as it is. This is the message you impart to her when you attempt to change her hair into something that goes against its curly nature. Teaching her that she is beautiful exactly the way she was born is a gift you will give her that will last the rest of her life.

It's so easy to get frustrated and yank through her tender curls. It's very tempting to want to try quick-fix solutions or the advice of well-meaning friends and family members who suggest chemical solutions that promise an easy combing. This usually backfires, however, because you will then need to contend with high-maintenance routines, broken hair, and, potentially, even second-degree burns. When very curly hair is combed through quickly, it's pulled from the scalp and it hurts—for some children, enough that they throw up from the stress and trauma of it. This pain establishes and reinforces the feeling that to have such hair means punishment and suffering; that something must be wrong with them for having such hair—when the opposite is true. Curls are joyful and spectacular. They are gifts that just need special care to show them in their best light. They need to be treated like fine silk, rather than simple and coarse wash-and-wear denim. When you know what curls want, they are no longer a big deal or a struggle. Embrace them and enjoy them. They are works of art that your child has grown.

All of the techniques in the book apply to children's hair, as well as to adults'. This is because we should always treat our curls as gently as if they were growing on a baby's head. For a rushed parent, however, it is good to have some step-by-step-instructions to comb a child's curls with as little pain as possible.

Here is a basic overview for how to make very curly baby hair more manageable. Afterward, I include advice on a few issues that may be faced by parents of very curly children, especially parents who have straighter hair than their children's (such as the parents of a mixed-race child, a transracially adopted child, or a foster child of African heritage). It's best if you follow these tips pretty closely. They all work together, and if you leave out one of the steps, your child's hair can still turn into a big fuzz ball. By following this advice, you will also have a baseline and will know what works for your child's hair; then, if you want to, you can experiment, always knowing you can fall back on these basic guidelines.

Step-by-Step Guide to Easy-Care Curls

This chapter will cover the seven simple steps to caring for your child's sweet curls that will help them last all week: shampoo, condition, comb, define, dry, protect, and refresh. Once you begin the process of washing and combing your child's curls, it's best to have everything you need nearby. These are the items I've found to make the process of washing and combing go more smoothly— if you have them ahead of time—before gathering up your little one to begin.

What You Will Need
- Enough time to let curls dry after washing and combing.
- A mild shampoo (see chapter 11 or TightlyCurly.com for product suggestions).
- Conditioner that is thick and *slippery*—but not sticky.
- A Denman-type brush (preferred) or a wide-toothed comb.
- A towel (to drape over the shoulders only).
- Clips (this is optional; they're used to hold back sections of hair that you have finished).
- Books or toys to keep a little one occupied.

Shampooing Little Curls

It's a good idea to wash a child's hair as early in the day as possible, to give her curls plenty of time to dry before bedtime.

When washing very curly hair, the goal is to keep the curls calm at all times (I will refer to the child as "her" for simplicity, but this applies equally to little boys—or to big ones, for that matter). Wash your little one's hair only about every four days to once a week. More often wears out her hair and is unnecessary unless she has gotten very dirty in the

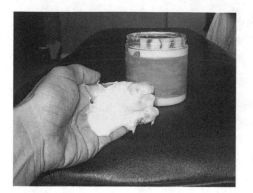

Put tons of thick, slippery conditioner in the hair.

meantime. It's better to do this in the morning so that her hair can dry for the rest of the day.

It's very important not to scrub or rub her hair, because this will mat it, in addition to being totally unnecessary. Scrubbing makes more work for you when you comb and damages her curls. When you wash, it's best to concentrate on her scalp. It's her scalp that needs the shampoo. When you rinse, shampoo will flow down her wet hair, and this is plenty.

Conditioning Little Curls

Apply *lots* of thick, slippery conditioner (see chapter 11 or TightlyCurly .com for recommendations). Use at least one generous handful if her hair is short and two for shoulder-length or longer hair. I use two heaping handfuls for my hair. It's also important to use the right conditioners. Some conditioners are *way* too light—they are little more than thickened water—and simply evaporate, leaving your child's hair defenseless. You need the real stuff to keep her curls calm (without being greasy, sticky, or crunchy). The type of conditioner you use is vital, but not in that it-has-to-cost-a-fortune way. Actually, I've found that many of the cheaper drug-store brands work best. Other brands are too light and simply evaporate, are too greasy, or build up and get sticky or crunchy.

Here is a big secret of giving your little one manageable hair: After putting in the conditioner, do not rinse it out. I know it sounds weird, but leave in that good conditioner. It has lots of work to do in your child's hair, and it can do its thing only when you leave it in. It weighs down tight curls and keeps them well defined and calm. Conditioner also weather-proofs her hair and keeps it moisturized. The right conditioner is your magic ingredient. Without the right conditioner, your child's hair may continue to puff up. Conditioner alone works better than gel because it keeps her curls defined without being crunchy, sticky, or drying, as gel can be.

Also, leaving in a good slippery conditioner makes a world of difference in your being able to get a comb or a Denman-type brush through her tight curls.

Combing Curls without Tears

It may be tempting to rub a towel into the child's curls to dry them, but it's best for both of you if you resist this urge. Rubbing a towel into curls mats them up and can easily damage them. (If ever there is a time you do need to remove excess water, however, gently dab her hair with the towel or softly press the towel to her hair without rubbing, then pick the towel up and move it to another spot to press again.) For the best combing experience, you need all of that water in her hair so that it stays wet as long as possible while you comb. You can put a towel over her shoulders to keep water from dripping down her back. You could use a spray bottle if her hair dries out as you comb it. (Try not to get the spray on her skin, though. It's cold and startling when it lands on delicate skin.) The reason for keeping her hair and the conditioner in her hair very wet is that it helps the comb or the Denman brush glide through her curls much more easily.

As you comb your child's hair, the hair responds best when it's soaking wet, with all of that good conditioner in it. Use a Denman-type brush (or a wide-toothed comb). The Denman is *not* the same as a bristle brush.

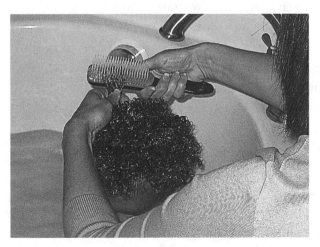

Grip the curls as you comb so that it doesn't hurt your child. Notice how Jennifer is firmly gripping Arden's hair between the scalp and where she is combing. This keeps the combing from hurting. In a very tangled or matted spot, she could give Arden's hair a couple of twists between her scalp and where she is combing and then pinch this between her fingers. If you use this Twist Pinch technique, your child will feel no pain and will probably play happily in the tub, even while her hair is being combed.

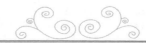

Too Much Conditioner?

If you have used the right amount of conditioner, it will foam up. Not to worry. It dries and disappears. You need lots of it in your child's hair to do the job. If any spot accumulates too much conditioner, just dab it with a little water when it dries. No big thing.

A regular bristle brush should never be used on tight curls. Denmans are more like a comb with several rows of teeth embedded in a rubber cushion. This means that the "give" when you comb comes from the Denman (or a Denman-type brush) and not from the delicate curls. Denman-type brushes put your child's curls together, whereas I've found that regular combs break curls apart.

To keep the combing from hurting, make sure you "pinch" her hair with your fingers between her scalp and where you are combing (see the photo on page 145). At a really tangled spot, give the section you're working on a couple of twists, then pinch it at the twist (as always, between her tender scalp and where you are combing) to avoid hurting your child. Believe me, it *hurts* to have curly hair combed without there being any barrier to the pain. If you can prevent the pain while combing, this will make the process less of an ordeal for both of you.

If she has lots of hair, you can work in bite-size sections. Comb out a section and clip it out of the way. This keeps a section you've finished from "visiting" the sections you are working on and getting tangled back up or caught in your comb.

Define the curls. Here Jennifer is twirling Arden's curls around her fingers. Another option is to run your fingers through the child's hair a few times. This helps all of her curls clump together, instead of each hair standing confused all on its own.

Define Those Curls

For a more manageable hairstyle that will last at least four days to a week, you need to define her curls. Otherwise, they clump and get confused or get fuzzy. You define the curls after her hair is combed with conditioner and while still wet. There are several methods you can use:

- You can gently run your hands through her hair a few times in the direction that her hair grows to separate it into individual curls.
- You can also take each curl and twirl it around your fingers for lots of stunning little "doodles"—as my mom calls them—or Shirley Temple curls (see chapter 6 for more photos and ideas on doodles). This also works wonderfully on a boy's or a man's curls.
- If you want more definition per curl and have enough time, take each curl that you see forming and run your fingers down it to smooth it. This method takes longer, but it creates perfect curls. This works best for hair that's about shoulder length or longer.

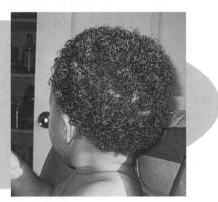

Let the curls dry with conditioner in them. This is Arden's hair while it dries. You can see that the conditioner is still visible. When you use enough product to give some weight to your child's curls, it will look white when wet. If there are still white gloppy sections after it dries, simply dab those parts with water, and they should disappear.

Let Curls Set: Drying

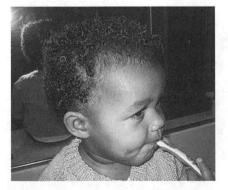

Wait for the curls to dry. This is Arden when her hair is totally dry.

For defined curls that last for days, they need time to set, much like pudding. From this moment on, don't comb, brush, or finger-comb your child's hair. Even finger-combing makes curls frizz up like a balloon. Pulling apart her curls makes them frizz. There is no way around this one. It may be tempting, but don't brush, comb, or finger-comb her hair again until the next time you wash it and have it soaking wet, with conditioner in it.

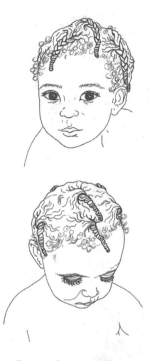

Protect hair at night. When her hair is long enough, you can put it into several braids or twists for bedtime.

Protect Little Curls

Unprotected curls rub against the pillow and can tangle, mat, and become damaged—not to mention harder to comb. By putting curls up at night in a calm and protective style (provided they are long enough to do this without pulling them tightly), hair remains smoother. To do this, wait until your child's curls have totally dried. Before bedtime, if her hair is long enough, put her curls in several braids, two-strand-twists, or buns to keep them smooth while she sleeps. For example, you could put two on top, one or two on each side, and one near the bottom. Braids or twists are better, but if you are using buns, try not to put one directly at the back of her head, because this can be uncomfortable. Putting curls up at night also works in a big way to calm them, which prevents her hair from tangling and getting all fuzzy and matted. There will also not be damage from bobby pins, with the hair rubbing against the metal of the pins if you braid or put her curls into twists instead.

If curls have had time to dry and set properly, they may look a little stringy or feel a bit stiff with the conditioner. This is good. It means your child's curls have set properly.

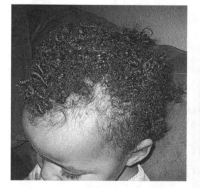

Take out the braids or the twists in the morning.

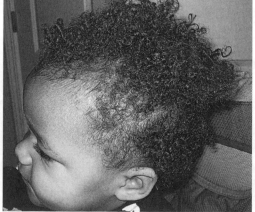

This is Arden in the morning, after her hair is taken out of its protective style. You can see that her hair is a bit tousled. This is easily fixable.

If there are any white patches after her hair has dried, simply dab them with water. By morning, her curls should be nice and soft, provided the right conditioner has been used.

Care between Washes: Refreshing Baby Curls

In the morning, unbraid or unbun your child's hair. At this point, it might look like an undefined mess and you may think that all of her curls are gone. They aren't. Curls may look smashed, undefined, fuzzy, or as if they escaped into the night. Those curls are still there; they're just sleeping. To wake them back up, smooth a little water and a bit more conditioner over her hair to calm any frizzies and refresh her curls. Resist the urge to finger-comb her hair while it's dry, though. Dry combing equals frizz. If you come to a tangled spot, you can wet that spot, dab a little conditioner on it, and then finger-comb that isolated troubled area. After you smooth it with water and conditioner (so that her hair is damp only), by the time it dries, her curls will be back and refreshed. You can twirl around your fingers any little doodles that got fuzzy, smashed, or uncoiled while she slept.

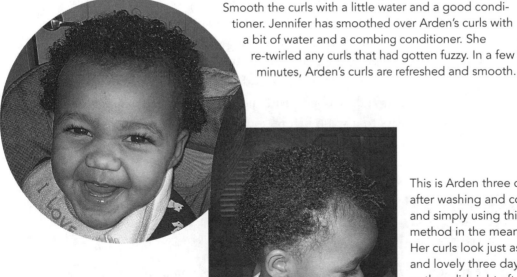

Smooth the curls with a little water and a good conditioner. Jennifer has smoothed over Arden's curls with a bit of water and a combing conditioner. She re-twirled any curls that had gotten fuzzy. In a few minutes, Arden's curls are refreshed and smooth.

This is Arden three days after washing and combing and simply using this method in the meantime. Her curls look just as smooth and lovely three days later as they did right after being washed and combed.

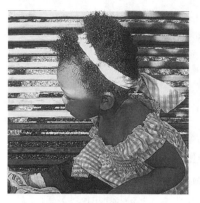

This is adorable Mya's hair before.

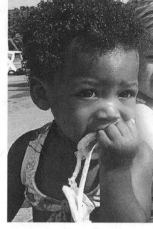

Although Mya's mom, Jencie, had done several things right, she was using a product that caused Mya's hair to become stiff and crunchy once it dried.

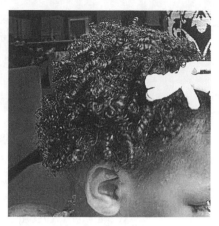

And this is Mya's hair after her hair is defined with doodles (see chapter 6), using one of the recommended conditioners. This style lasts about four days, even after getting wet. Her lovely spirals look so natural that people have come up to ask whether her hair is naturally curly.

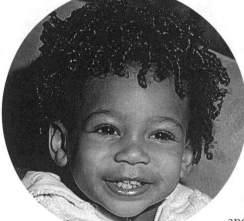

Mya several months later. You can see that her hair is already growing and looks glossy and healthy.

It's fine if your child's hair is too short to braid. Simply have her sleep on her hair the way it is now, and in the morning smooth over it as often as needed, keeping your hands wet with water and a little conditioner. Add a bit more conditioner if her hair really frizzes. This should get rid of morning fuzziness and smashed curls. These curls should last about four days to a week before you need to wash, condition, and comb them again.

Do I Need to Use Products Made Specifically for Little Ones?

The most important qualities in a product you use on a child are that it doesn't irritate and that it helps you cleanse and comb her hair in the gentlest way possible, depending on whether it's a shampoo or a conditioner. You don't have to use a product that is meant only for kids. A good product works well for everyone. For manageable curls, it's important to leave in the conditioner. Yet it's just as crucial to use the right kind of conditioner. Not all conditioners that market themselves for children will work with this technique. For example, conditioners that are too light will evaporate as if they were never there, and conditioners that are stiff or sticky can build up and make hair stiff or sticky and difficult to manage.

Especially for little ones (who tend to have more sensitive skin), it's best to avoid products with fragrances and essential oils, extracts, or botanical infusions, because these can irritate the skin. In particular, avoid any product with mint, menthol, cinnamon, or citrus, such as lime, lemon, or even orange. Just think about how much those substances can burn if you get them into a cut. They're stronger than you might think. Fragrances are usually listed near the bottom of the ingredients list (see chapter 11 for more information on ingredients and products, or TightlyCurly.com). Essential oils and extracts can appear anywhere on the label, however, even near the top as infusions. Scented oils and extracts are different from unscented oils like coconut, olive, jojoba, or shea butter, which are desired moisturizing ingredients.

Although many great products and companies are out there, some companies rely on old wives' tales and consumer fears to spread misinformation about ingredients that have actually been proven to be very safe. For delicate skin, it's more important that products don't cause irritation. Some conditioners may not be slippery enough to enable you to get a comb through tight curls. When the hair isn't slippery enough, forcing and yanking a comb through it causes damage, as well as severe pain. Some conditioners are too light, and after all of your hard work combing and defining the curls, the conditioners may evaporate, leaving your little one's curls puffy instead of smooth and defined.

There are many definitions of what makes a product natural. Some products say they're natural—and then charge high prices for saying so—but in reality they often use nearly the same working ingredients as less expensive conditioners. They may simply throw in a few extra exotic-sounding plant extracts. Always beware of products that aren't moisturizing or slippery enough to help you comb tightly curly hair (even though they might say they are). There are wonderful, helpful ingredients in affordably priced products found in drugstores, as well as in natural products. Keep in mind that "natural" doesn't always equal safe. Many products add exotic and essential oils, which tend to be highly irritating to sensitive skin (even some that say fragrance-free).

Styles for Little Curls

Here are a few easy styles for children that keep their curls safe while they play. I know I keep saying this, but you never want to brush, comb, or finger-comb dry curls, not even to put the child's hair in these styles; otherwise, you will end up with a damaged puff ball. A little water and conditioner smoothed over any fuzzy spots will work beautifully.

What You Need to Style Your Child's Curls
- Water
- A combing conditioner (see chapter 11 or TightlyCurly.com for product suggestions)
- A fabric-covered band or plastic clips, depending on the hairstyle

You Do Not Need
- A brush
- A comb

You can easily smooth wild morning curls into a nice, easy style. Simply wet your hands, add a little combing conditioner, rub your hands together, and run them over her fuzzy parts. Repeat as needed, adding a bit of water and/or combing conditioner when necessary. I've found that styles requiring lots of sectioning, such as French braids or cornrows, are not a good option. Not only are they time consuming to do, but they can damage curls when the hair is sectioned, pulled apart, and combed. This also really hurts the child's scalp when it's done in a hurry.

Here are some style ideas:

- You can put her hair in one or two low braids. (With hair as curly as hers, you can simply braid it to the ends and leave it—no bands or clips are needed at all. Generally, her curls will happily stay braided. If necessary, you can wet the ends, put in a bit of conditioner, and twirl the ends of her braids around your fingers to "seal" them for the day. Otherwise, if her hair is long enough, you can stop near the ends. Tight curls usually stay braided or twisted together until they're undone. It's often the unbraiding that's a challenge. Yet it's not hard to undo braids if you employ a few tricks and patience: to unbraid, smooth over her braided ends with a bit of water and conditioner, and that should make it easier. A time-saving bonus with braids: your child could sleep in this style—I often do—and in the morning simply smooth over any fuzzy parts, as well as her ends, with more water and conditioner. This saves not only time, but wear and tear on her hair. For variety, you could undo half of the braids so that they have really curly ends—this is very cute.)
- You could put her hair in one or two low buns. (Goody makes some great hair pins—see chapter 11 for a picture of what these bun clips look like.)
- You could put her hair in one or two braids, then twist the braids into a bun or buns—using the same hair pins mentioned earlier to anchor them. When they're finished, they appear way more complicated than they actually are to do.
- You can put her hair in two low ponytails. I've found that when I smooth and define my curls, my hair just naturally parts right down the center without my having to do a thing. If this is true for your daughter, then you can simply take half of her hair, put a fabric-coated rubber band around it, then do the other half. It's best not to double the band. Her curls will keep the band in place. If you twist the band into her hair, it will damage it, as well as snarl in her curls so badly that you may have to cut it out of her hair.
- Make double buns. Divide her hair in half from ear to ear so that you end up with a top half and a bottom half. Take the top half, twirl

it into a bun, and pin it. Do the same with the bottom half so that the buns are on top of each other. It's adorable to leave out the ends to show the little spirals peeking out.

- You could gently pin back the top half of her hair in a clip, with the bottom half down.

These are the basics of several easy styles that are gentle on hair (as long as the rubber band is loose in your child's hair for the ponytail styles). For more style ideas and for photos and step-by-step illustrations on how to create these styles, check out chapter 13.

For Brand New Ones: Let Baby Hair Be

While your little one still has baby hair, it's best to gently rinse her hair in warm water or delicately wipe over her hair with a soft, wet, warm wash-cloth. (You may want to test the water's temperature as you would a bottle's by running or dabbing it on the inside of your arm.)

You can begin the techniques in this chapter (and this book) as soon as your child's real curls come in. At first, you might simply want to finger-comb and smooth her hair after washing it (no Denman brush), because her scalp is so delicate. When her hair needs more combing than your fingers can do, very gently use the Denman or a comb, being careful to avoid her scalp until she is older and her scalp isn't as delicate.

With hair so new, you don't need to put it up when she sleeps—only do this when it starts to get longer and tangly. Pulling hair tight, especially on a child this young, is unnecessary, and it can hurt her tender scalp if she sleeps on bobby pins or clips or her hair is pulled at the roots. Wait until the hair is longer, long enough to get tangled. You can leave her hair alone until there are enough curls that need help in staying calm.

You shouldn't need to do much trimming or cutting of a little one's hair. The only time this may be needed is if her hair has grown in notice-ably different lengths (baby hair often comes in in patches, and these are best left alone to grow in as the hair wants, until all of it has come in).

If it turns out that you do need to trim to even out her hair—or, for a boy—to keep it in a shorter style, you may be able to trim it yourself. This is a possibility only as long as she always wears it curly (curls are forgiving; straight hair isn't). For more detailed instructions on trimming, look over the steps in chapter 7.

Should I . . .?

There will be many people who feel that they have the best advice for your child—especially if you are a new mom who is not yet familiar with taking care of very curly hair. Well-meaning in-laws, friends, or even strangers may try to pressure you into believing certain old wives' tales about caring for very curly hair. Following are some of the worst myths.

Chemicals

By chemicals, I mean anything that permanently alters the texture of curls (until new hair grows in) even if the hair-care item is advertised as being natural or for kids. These products include relaxers, texturizers, kiddie perms, textulaxers, kiddie texturizers, naturlaxers, or any other clever and misleading word play. Because you are reading this, I know you want to care for your little one's beautiful curls as they are. I hope what I'm about to say will fortify you against well-meaning strangers, beauticians, friends, in-laws, and family members who suggest that you "do something" about those innocent and joyful natural curls—meaning, "make her hair conform." Many people have it set in their minds from a very young age that tight curls are something to be broken or "cured." I have found that what our curls need is the freedom to be their own happy selves.

Take it from a child who grew up with her hair cared for in both black and white households that the best thing you can do is help a child learn what works for her natural curls. I spent my childhood, adolescence, and young adulthood applying chemicals to my hair because that was what I'd been taught. It never did me any good when I tried to force my hair into being a poor and broken imitation of other people's straighter hair. Yet my hair has blossomed and grown once I put down the chemicals and embraced the curls I was born with.

Anything strong enough to permanently change the shape of hair is a harsh chemical. It takes powerful chemicals to break the bonds of our hair in order to reshape it. Some products may call themselves natural, but always remember that not all natural things are safe or gentle. For example, consider arsenic, hemlock, mercury, and venoms made by certain snakes, spiders, and box jellyfish. If a product is powerful enough to break the strong bonds in the hair to change its shape, it's too corrosive for your, or your child's, delicate hair. These products usually contain a highly alkaline, caustic base and sometimes also have an acid to finish off the work (for more information on what happens when chemicals are put on hair, see chapter 12). These chemicals are scary, no matter how familiar they may feel or how happy the model looks on the box. Too often, they cause unbearable pain and can leave second-degree burns in their wake.

But beyond all this, you never want to give a child the message that you would take the chance of burning her—or would actually burn her—with lye-type chemicals, rather than deal with the hair she was born with.

"Training"

This makes me shudder. It is perhaps the second most harmful thing to do to a child's tender scalp, after perms. It's a myth that curly hair needs to be "trained" by pulling it back or up tightly, so that a child can get used to it. There is no reason in the world that a baby or a child should ever have to get used to something that hurts her and can cause long-term damage. Pulling hair tightly and constantly can cause traction alopecia. Traction alopecia occurs as a result of constant stress on, and the pulling of, the hair's follicles to the point that they no longer function. Soon they are damaged beyond repair, and those spots become very thin, patchy, or even bald. Sometimes the follicles can recover and growth will resume if the pulling stops, but in other cases, the damage is permanent. There is no reason to do this to a child (or to anyone, for that matter). Curly hair will grow and thrive if you use the very gentle techniques described in this book. Hair care should never hurt anyone. If it hurts, it means something is being done wrong.

Extensions

Believe it or not, some people may suggest putting additional hair in your child's hair, with extensions or weaves. Apart from this sending a message to your child that you prefer store-bought hair over the child's own, this can harm her scalp in the same way that "training" can. This is because the child's delicate roots must support the extra weight of the hair, in addition to stress from the tight styles that her real hair is put in to support the stranger's hair. Wearing extensions and weaves can also cause traction alopecia, which may result in permanent damage.

Oiling the Scalp

Another myth is that oiling the scalp is healthy and can help hair grow. A buildup of thick, heavy oils and greases on the scalp will actually clog and damage the follicles. If your child has a dry scalp, it may be that her hair is being washed too often, the shampoo might be too harsh or may not be getting rinsed out well enough, or the conditioner isn't moisturizing enough.

Before you resort to using oils, first try smoothing a little of the rinsing conditioner over her hair (if you are doing this step—see chapter 3), This should be plenty. If her scalp still seems dry or if it is flaking, have your child checked by her doctor, just to make sure the dryness doesn't have an underlying cause.

If none of these things is the case, then it's okay to put a *very* light coating of a natural liquid oil on the scalp. You can do this by putting a dime-size drop in your hands, rubbing your hands together, and smoothing it gently over her scalp. This insures that only the very lightest amount of oil—just enough to counteract any dryness—is used. However, it's best to do this as infrequently as possible, such as only once a week, perhaps after washing, combing, defining, and drying her hair.

Your Gift of Understanding

Your little one is unique and has the hair to prove it. If you were born with wavy or straighter hair than your child was, hair may not seem like a big deal to you. This makes sense because you most likely have been able to run a comb through your hair without giving it much thought and can go swimming without worrying about what to do with your hair. In addition, the attributes of your hair have been reflected and affirmed back to you in nearly every type of media you have been exposed to since you were young.

The wonderful thing is that a child with very curly hair never has to hate her hair. Because you are reading this, you're taking the necessary steps for her to be comfortable in her own body and with her natural hair. You have the power to prevent a child from going through any trauma associated with curly hair. Tightly curly hair is like no other kind of hair. It needs totally different care from all other hair types. Once you know what it needs, however, it will thrive, and its care is no longer a challenge or an issue.

Curls will always take a bit longer to care for than straighter hair does, but I feel that the rewards for understanding it are far greater as well. The greater rewards come not only from your child's escaping the pain and feelings of self-hate that she can internalize surrounding her hair, but from her experiencing the peace of not having to worry all the time about her hair. I tell you, there is nothing like a child with a head full of happy curls—they seem to radiate joy to the tips. If a child is loved and accepted totally, including her hair, this will last the rest of her life. You can help a child understand that her hair is wonderful and wondrous, that it's worth the time to care for properly (and without pain), and that you wouldn't change a thing about her. She has the right to enter adulthood not only knowing how to care for her own hair, but also knowing that it is beautiful. You are able to send her into the rest of her life at peace with herself, so that her time and energy can be channeled into bigger issues in her life.

The goal, I have discovered (as one who owns such tightly curly hair), is for your child to grow up feeling that hair is *not* a big deal.

TAKE AWAY Tips

- It's best to use products with as little fragrance and as few colors as possible. These can irritate sensitive skin.

- As with all curls, handle your child's curls gently. (Curls are silk, not denim.)

- Always pinch hair between where you are combing and the child's sensitive scalp. Combing tight curls roughly hurts!

- Never style your child's hair in ways that pull tightly or that smother her tender scalp. This can permanently damage her hair follicles.

- Never use harsh chemicals or extreme heat on a child's hair.

- By teaching your child that her hair is beautiful exactly as it grows from her head, you will be giving her a gift of self-acceptance that will last the rest of her life.

Chapter Nine

Highlights
Do-It-Yourself Tips

In my teenage years, among my other hair experiments, I bought highlighter kits. They always included a little plastic cap with holes in it. You were supposed to pull the strands of hair you'd selected for highlighting through the holes, using the plastic crochet hook that came with the kit. I could never get my hair through those darn holes. My chosen strands wouldn't want to separate from their neighbor hairs, so when I tried to pull a few of them out, they brought all of the surrounding hairs with them. I'd end up having to take off the cap and fight apart every section of hair. By the time I'd gotten my hair through the holes, the holes were stretched open and torn. My hair beneath the cap was now a swarm of tangles, and my head throbbed from the tugging. If your hair is very curly, a highlighter cap probably won't work for you either.

If you're like me, you might not feel comfortable in the hands of a hairdresser, who might rip a comb through your coils in record time or otherwise rush the process in ways that damage your hair. So, you may want to try highlighting your hair on your own. Highlights, when done properly, emphasize your curls by making a few of them stand out against the others. This showcases the intricate and quirky twists that make your hair unique. Plus, you save money by doing this yourself.

I recommend that you read the entire highlighting chapter before you start the procedure, to ensure that everything makes sense. My suggestions are probably a little different from the directions that are included in regular highlighting kits, because mine are adjusted for tight curls.

What to Buy

The key to creating good highlights is to keep your hair looking as natural as possible. Anything radical should be left to more experienced hands. Your highlights should be only a few shades lighter than your natural color. That's why I use regular hair-coloring kits in a shade a bit lighter than my own. I don't buy streaking or highlighting kits because the range of colors is narrow, and the choices are usually too harsh and too light for my dark hair. If your hair is lighter, however, these might be an option for you.

It can be overwhelming to choose a color when you're standing in the drugstore, surrounded by dozens of nearly the same shades. The easiest way to choose a color is to match the shade that's closest to your ends. If your hair is long, your ends are probably several shades lighter than the hair at your scalp. I hold up a handful of my ends. Then I go from box to box, flopping my ends down on each picture to compare them. I do this until I find a good match. Or I wrangle my mother to help me choose a color that matches my ends. If your hair is dark, you might also want to try a hair color that is meant for dark hair.

What You'll Need
- A highlighter kit or a hair-coloring kit
- An old towel you don't mind getting stained

- Petroleum jelly to protect your scalp and hairline
- Plastic wrap to protect the rest of your hair
- Clips or bobby pins to hold the plastic wrap in place and to hold the selected hair strands you'll be highlighting
- Plastic measuring spoons (to measure out smaller quantities of the product, if desired)
- A cheap plastic container to mix smaller amounts of the product
- A plastic spoon to stir the mixture
- A timer
- Paper towels to clean up any spills
- Something to entertain yourself with for the twenty or so minutes it takes the process to work

The best strategy for creating natural-looking highlights is to choose about twenty to thirty strands, here and there, from approximately a dozen curls on your head. Don't do an entire curl unless the color you've chosen is very close to your own color. When you sprinkle glimmering strands throughout your hair, you make it shimmer. This is better than having bold stripes of color laid over your hair that look like twisty landing strips.

The best way to get your strands where you need them is to highlight on the day you're washing and combing your hair anyway. Highlight before you wash your hair. Choose the curl you'd like to add some shimmer to and patiently finger-comb it apart, always starting at the ends. Then select a pinch of hairs you'd like to highlight and pin them off to the side, out of the way. Pin the rest of your curl up somewhere safe. Do this to all of your selected curls until you've amassed a pile of hair to be highlighted.

When all of your sections are ready, apply petroleum jelly to your hairline and scalp. Also, put some around the base of any hairs you don't want colored but that might be in danger of having color fall on them. Do your strand test (very important!), and follow the product's directions from that point on. You can use plastic wrap as a barrier to protect the top of your hair, if necessary. I bobby pin or clip the plastic wrap in place around my head, working around the pieces of hair to be colored, so that they stick out of the plastic. When you have finished highlighting, be sure to rinse your highlighted hair thoroughly.

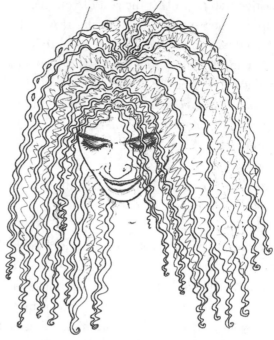

Highlights placed throughout the hair

For natural looking high-lights: If you highlight whole curls, go only slightly lighter than your natural color. If you high-light smaller amounts (about twenty hairs per section), it's okay to go a bit brighter.

If I make a mistake, I can always go back to the store, get another box of color that matches my own, and apply it—*only* to any place I messed up on. Now you can wash, condition, and comb your hair after highlight-ing it, to wash out the petroleum jelly and any remaining highlighting liquid. When you comb your hair, your highlights will be incorporated back into your curls, so you'll have little glimmers running through some of your curls. Not too many, but enough to make them special.

Why Highlights Only?

I suggest highlights instead of coloring your entire head to minimize the damage caused by lightening your hair. When you select a few curls to lighten, only those will be damaged from the hydroxide and the peroxide (see chapter 12). If your whole head is lightened, then all of your hair will be damaged. This could make it more time consuming to comb, may cause more matting, and eventually might result in breakage. By restricting the chemicals to a select few spots, if this process damages your hair, it will be only a tiny portion of your hair. The rest of your hair will still be virgin hair and will continue to be healthy.

This is what I've done. I wanted a few highlights to emphasize my curls but in no way wanted an entire head of damaged hair. So I chose about ten small sections of hair around my hairline and lightened only those to match the natural color at the ends.

Short Hair Exception

If you have short hair and you don't want to grow it long, you can color all of your hair at once. You can even color it drastically if you have natural curls and you're keeping your hair very short. Why? Because damage will break your hair and keep it short. If you wanted short hair in the first place, it won't matter that much. Plus, combing will be easy because your hair is short, so even if it tangles a bit more because of any damage, you still won't need much time to get a comb through it.

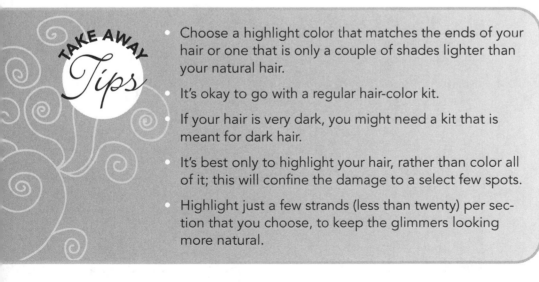

TAKE AWAY Tips

- Choose a highlight color that matches the ends of your hair or one that is only a couple of shades lighter than your natural hair.

- It's okay to go with a regular hair-color kit.

- If your hair is very dark, you might need a kit that is meant for dark hair.

- It's best only to highlight your hair, rather than color all of it; this will confine the damage to a select few spots.

- Highlight just a few strands (less than twenty) per section that you choose, to keep the glimmers looking more natural.

Chapter Ten

After the Chemicals and Severe Damage
Sometimes You Have to Walk through the Fire

I t can be scary to consider growing out a perm, especially if you haven't seen the natural texture of your hair since babyhood—if ever. I've found that the only way to have long, healthy hair is to avoid using all of the lye-type chemicals and to deal only with virgin hair. Those chemicals are toxic to your hair. They are composed of the same ingredients as hair depilatories. The only difference is that relaxers are (hopefully) rinsed out before they completely dissolve your hair, while depilatories stay on a little longer to finish the job. There's no way any ingredient that is strong enough to rearrange the very bonds that hold your hair together can be anything but damaging (see chapter 12).

Treat this time of new growth as special, and cherish it. You are

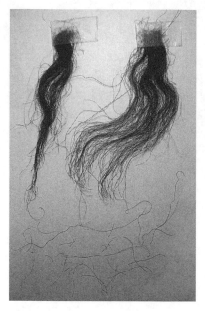

These are the last two pieces of my chemically damaged hair after I cut it off. I taped them into a book. Years later, even protected within the pages of the book, they continue to break apart.

giving birth to a whole new head of hair. Remember this time, take photographs, write about your experiences, and become acquainted with this beautiful new part of yourself that you are discovering. There is a purity and a simplicity to wearing your own true curls. There is a calmness in being and accepting all of who you are as a whole person.

Your body is in the process of creating. It is making something just for you. It's like watching wildflower seeds grow in earth that was once burned by fire. You are watching new life swell from a place where once everything was scorched. I do have to say that cutting off my relaxed hair (when I was ready) was and continues to be the best gift I could have given myself. It was my first giant leap toward finally making peace with the hair I had and all of the mental baggage I'd been carrying around regarding my hair. You might not know what a treasure you have in your hair until you can face it as it is, learn about it, accept it, and grow to love it fiercely.

Your Two Textures

Although cutting off the chemically damaged hair and starting fresh is much easier than living with it as it gradually grows out, it might be too much of a leap for you just yet. Growing your hair out, which I chose to do, although absolutely worth it, is a struggle. The areas where your chemically damaged hair is joined to the new growth will mat as if it's been turned into quilt batting. I've heard this matted area referred to as "scab hair." Scab hair is a perfect way of thinking about this band of matting (if it happens to you as it did to me). While your whole head of hair is "healing" from the damaging chemicals, there will often be a band that marks the place where the healthy new hair is still connected to the damaged, chemically altered hair. Know that, like a scab, this is part of the process of growing out the damage and starting fresh.

When I was growing out my relaxer, I let my hair grow for about a year and a half before I was ready to cut off the chemically damaged part. To match the two textures of my hair (my curly roots versus the crunchy, straighter, relaxed hair), after I washed and combed my hair I set it in about twenty two-strand twists (I'll show you how to make these twists later in the chapter). This process took me about three hours every week. I spent most of the time trying to get the comb through the mats that formed against my scalp, especially at the top-back of my head. I worried that the mats were my new growth coming in, and that this was what my entire head would be like when I cut off the chemically damaged hair.

To my relief, I found out that wasn't the case. The mats were happening where the yin and the yang of my two radically different hair types were joined. Because the textures were so different, whenever they touched each other on the same strands of hair, they created a perfect storm of matting. As time passed, the mats traveled down my hair as my new growth got longer. Once I cut off the chemically ruined hair, I never had matting like that again. When you first start to grow out the chemicals, you might think your new growth is causing the mat at your hairline. It's not. The matting is caused by the connection point where the damaged hair changes into the healthy hair. These are two totally different creatures, and their yin-yang characteristics cause them to mat where they are joined together.

During the growing-out period, the majority of the tips I suggest in this book, such as leaving in the conditioner and separating your curls, might not work for processed hair. These techniques are intended to reinforce and work with your hair's natural curl. Because your hair might have had most or all of its curl stripped out, the advice might not work as well for you until your chemically damaged hair is gone. Once the old, processed, and broken hair has been cut off, however, you can use these techniques to encourage and support your new growth. What this means is that if you choose to leave the processed hair attached to your new hair, you'll have to use alternative styling methods until you're ready to cut off the damaged hair.

Your New Hair

When you first cut off the chemically ravaged hair, you're left with new short hair. Your hair will grow outward, rather than down, for a while. And it might seem like your hair is expanding out like spray foam as it grows, but this is both the frustration and the wonder of our curls. Enjoy this time of getting acquainted with the true beauty of your natural coils. Also, enjoy the freedom of this hair. Right after you cut your hair short, it will be much easier to wash and comb it, and it won't be much work to comb it after swimming. You might enjoy this hair so much you may decide to keep it at this wash-and-go length.

As your hair gets longer, the spirals at the ends will begin to weigh down the rest of your hair. At some point, a critical mass will be reached. This is when your hair is long enough to weigh itself down. When this tipping point occurs, your hair will grow down instead of out. Leaving in

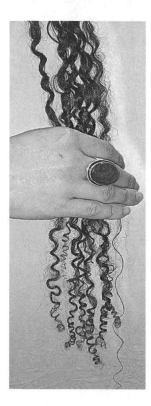

conditioner and dividing and smoothing each curl will help your curls stay nicely clumped together. If you're impatient to see some length, using conditioner this way will also make the growing-down instead of growing-out stage happen faster. This is because you're adding weight to your curls. The ends of my hair are in tight spirals, slightly smaller than the diameter of a pencil, about one-fourth inch across. These little coils weigh the rest of my hair down like fishing sinkers. Because my hair is also very long, there's lots of weight to pull it down.

The longer your hair, the looser your curls will begin to look at your scalp. For example, if you followed my curls from beginning to end, you'd see that they go from nearly straight at my scalp to wavy, to curly in the middle, to tightly coiled at the ends.

If I were to cut my hair short, I'd have an Afro until it grew long enough to weigh itself down again. It's funny: when I was young, I had no idea that the best way to get long hair would be to stop using all of the chemicals and embrace my curls.

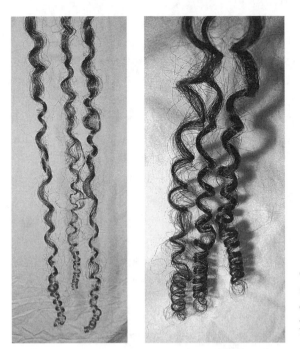

Compare these curls to the mug shot of my chemically damaged locks from many years ago (shown at the beginning of this chapter).

Setting Your Two Textures while Growing Out the Chemicals

There are several ways to set your hair so that its two textures appear uniform until you're ready to cut off the perm-damaged hair. The two-stranded twist is an excellent solution. You can also use braids to keep the two different textures of your hair looking similar.

For either set, start by washing and conditioning your hair. Leave only a little conditioner in your hair in this case, because relaxed hair can't soak in much conditioner. Separate out a section that you want to work on (the size depends on whether you're doing twists or braids; see the following section), and pin back the rest of your hair. Comb this section, then squeeze it gently in a towel to remove the extra water. Your hair should be barely damp, because air can't get in to dry your hair as easily when it's set as when it's loose. Blotting the water out of your hair gives it a jump-start on drying.

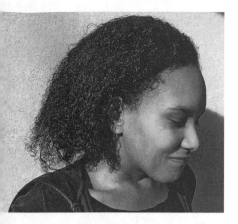

This is gorgeous Brianna. Her hair has been damaged by the frequent use of a flat iron to the point that her hair no longer forms curls.

Twists

Divide the freshly combed area into one- to two-inch-square sections. Divide each section in half, and twist one half around the other down to the ends. When you get to the bottom, twirl the ends back together to form a single curl. If the ends have dried, wet them, dab a little conditioner on them, and twist them around your finger. Put this twist back into a clip, and start again with another section. Very curly hair will do better with smaller twists, because smaller twists make tighter wave patterns. If your hair is less curly, you could get away with bigger twists, because they will make looser waves. Sleep in the twists, and remove them only when they're totally dry.

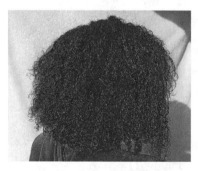

Brianna's hair from the back.

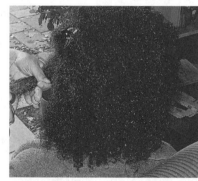

To grow out her hair without cutting off all the damage, she can match the texture of her new growth and the damaged growth by putting in twists (you can also use braids or French braids for a similar effect). We started by separating her freshly washed and conditioned hair into about one-inch sections and combing it.

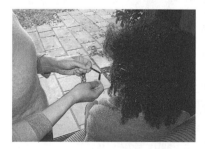

After combing out the tangles, I divided every section in half and twisted it to the ends.

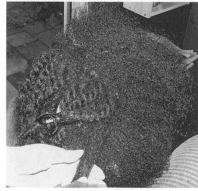

As each section is twisted, it's clipped out of the way. Her hair is spritzed, and more combing conditioner is added when the hair begins to dry out.

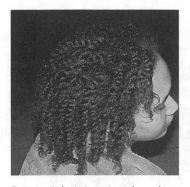

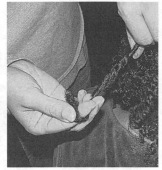

Brianna's hair is twisted, and we wait for it to dry. The best thing to do is sleep on the twists and undo them in the morning. This gives you a firm set that can last all week. If you need your hair to dry faster, you can use a hair dryer on a low setting. Always check the temperature; if it burns your skin, it's way too hot for your hair.

When the twists are dry, untwist them. I hold the ends and untwist them open from the bottom by twirling them until they are loose. Then, with my other hand, I gently open them from the top, still holding onto the ends to keep them from snarling. As I hold them, I continue to twirl them until they open.

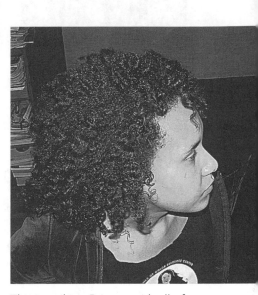

This is striking Brianna with all of her twists out. Her hair has much more definition. This style is great to hide the two textures while you grow out your hair until you're ready to cut off the damaged parts.

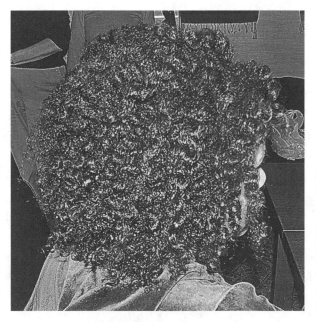

Brianna's hair from the back. (Brianna was a trooper. Before her hair had a chance to dry, the neighborhood had a power outage. We ended up taking her finished photos in total darkness, by aiming the camera in her direction and shooting with a flash. I didn't see her hair at this stage until the photos were developed several days later.)

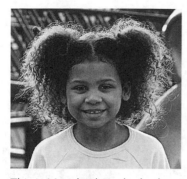

This is Mariah when she had a texturizer in her hair. Notice how frazzled her hair looks from the chemicals (it looks just like mine did when I used a texturizer).

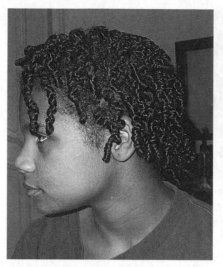

Mariah, after her mom, April, cut off the damaged parts and began to twist her hair in two-strand twists after washing and combing it.

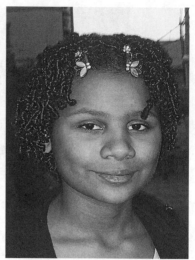

Gorgeous Mariah with her twists undone and lovely clips holding her hair out of her face. Notice how glossy and collected her curls look now.

Braids

Divide your hair into larger sections. You could go with three or four braids for each half of your hair, depending on its length. You'll need more braids for shorter hair so that all of your hair can make it into a braid. Your hair should be slightly damp to nearly dry. Apply only a little conditioner to moisturize; as mentioned earlier, relaxed hair can't soak it up very well. (The best method I've found is to let the section dry out before you braid it, then mist it lightly with water.)

Because your hair should be nearly dry (air has a very hard time getting inside your braids to dry them), you need to treat your hair carefully. Once you've braided your hair to the bottom, you can finish with a twist if your permed hair still has some curl (see the night braid photo in chapter 7). If it doesn't, braid it to the ends to hold it. Let this set all night or until it's totally dry. The next day, unbraid your hair. Fluff it lightly with your fingers to break apart the braid pattern.

After the Chop

It takes courage to make a big change like chopping off the chemically treated hair, but having your own true hair is worth it. When I did it, I was amazed at how differently my new hair felt from the old hair. My new hair was soft, shiny, and smooth—a radical departure from the dry, rough, and dull hair I'd spent my whole life, up until then, believing was my "real" hair.

Doodles

When you first cut off the chemically damaged hair, if you have cut your hair very short, you could set your hair with doodles. This emphasizes each curl and helps rein-force them when they're too short to separate by running your hands down each curl. After wash-ing your hair and leaving conditioner in it, take each curl and twist it around your finger. This will make lots of little mini–Shirley Temple twists all over your head. This styling will cut down on fuzz for the strands of hair that have a hard time finding a curl to belong to; twisting the fuzzies into nearby curls reinforces, as well as defines, each curl. My mother wears her hair in this striking style and gets compliments from strangers and coworkers all the time. (For more examples of doodles, see Aja's and Frances's lovely curls in chapter 6.)

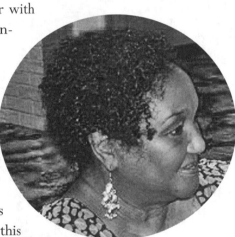

This is a photo of my mom with her doodles, right after we cut her hair short.

Other Ideas

The basic smoothing techniques recommended in chapter 6 also work well for shorter hair. If your curls are looser, you could run your fingers through your curls when they're wet with conditioner. This helps to sep-arate and define them.

It took about ten years after the Big Chop for my natural short hair to grow long enough to reach down to my hips. Growing out the chemically ruined hair isn't easy, but it will be the best thing you could ever do for your hair. And it will free you. You'll know that you are all *you*. There won't be any monsters hiding under the bed of your hair, so to speak. Giving up hair-damaging chemicals is like looking under the bed and discovering that the shadows you didn't want to face were actually hiding a new friend—a friend who will help you become even more comfortable in your own skin for having set it free.

TAKE AWAY Tips

- You might have matting where the two textures of your hair meet. If you aren't ready to chop, camouflage your two textures with twists or braids.

- The Big Chop takes a giant leap of faith, but it's worth it.

- Our hair keeps growing, giving us yet one more chance to finally do right by it.

- Have patience. You are giving birth to an entirely new head of hair, as well as a new relationship to it.

- Cherish this time, and remember it. Something wonderful is happening before your eyes.

- Natural hair is a gift we give to ourselves that keeps getting better over time.

Chapter Eleven

Your Toolbox
The Best Products and Tools for Your Hair

During junior high and into adulthood, I was an avid product label reader. I had no idea what any of the ingredients meant. All I knew was that nothing I'd tried so far had helped my hair, so I scanned the labels looking for ingredients I hadn't tried before, hoping I'd find the one that worked. One product that I desperately wanted to work was a favorite hairdressing made of all-natural ingredients. I loved that you could see the herbs ground up and suspended within the product. I used it for years. It smelled really good, too. Yet even though I used it every night, my hair just kept breaking off as if every strand were dotted with tear-off perforations.

Too often, we look to products to help "cure" the damage that was done to our hair. It's easy to get misled by companies presenting products that claim to "repair" hair. Although we know better, some of the ads are very convincing. It would be so nice if all we had to do was find magical products to use, and we could grow long, flowing hair with little effort. My stepmom, Ruth, told me a story about working in a community garden many years ago that illustrates this all-too-human failing. Ruth, an avid gardener, works hard to grow magnificent gardens that burst with happy plants and vegetables. While her garden plot in this communal garden was thriving, a fellow gardener was struggling with his plot. Every so often, he asked her how she got such an amazing garden: Was it a particular brand of fertilizer? What product did she use to make it grow like that? And Ruth said she always started to tell him exactly what she did to have such an abundant garden: "First, you dig a really deep hole. Then you fill it with lots of good, rich compost. Then—" And at this point the man usually cut her off, saying, "No, no, I mean what *product* do you use?" He didn't want to hear about the continued effort and mindful care she put into making her garden thrive. He wanted the one easy miracle product that would require no work on his part. He didn't want to hear about the hard work she put into the earth from day one to get such growth. And it's the same with our hair. It takes time, care, patience, and thought to grow beautiful hair. There are no miracle products; however, the right hair-care products are tools that make taking care of our hair easier—much as the right shovel, trowel, or twist-tie can help us work and manage a bountiful garden.

If we understand our hair, we'll be able to make informed, realistic decisions on its behalf. Knowing what a product can do—and what it can't—is like wearing a pair of truth-vision glasses when we flip over a bottle and read its label. Products usually exaggerate what they can do for your hair, so they're often misleading. The only place a product is legally bound to tell you the truth is in its list of ingredients. Once we know how to translate the ingredients, we will know whether it's our friend or foe. This chapter gives an overview of the best ingredients for your tight curls, tips on how to choose products and tools that work for your hair, and a few recommendations to get you started. If you're curious why I chose these products or you have questions about their ingredients, I explain what makes them work so well for tight curls in the "How to Choose the Best Products for Your Hair" section, under "Choosing Conditioners: The Best Ingredients to Look For." You can also check out what various ingredients actually do in the ingredients dictionary at TightlyCurly.com.

Recommended Shampoos and Conditioners for Your Curls

The following recommendations are in no way exhaustive, but they give you a nice sampling of different types of products in a reasonable price range that work for super-curly hair. I'm sure there are plenty of other products out there that might work as well for your hair. I'm also aware that leaving conditioner in your hair isn't glamorous or might seem too simple, but it works. I say, why pay twice as much or more for other products that, at best, do what conditioner already does? Personally, I usually alternate between two brands of products at any one time, so you don't have to have a large collection of bottles lining your sink. Find a couple of products that work for you, and that's plenty.

Conditioners are far more important for your hair than shampoos are. Conditioners are the workhorses for your curls. Because they perform so many duties, it's best to pick the ones that excel in the crucial areas. Leaving conditioner in your hair won't work if you have one that builds up in your hair or is so watery that it evaporates as if you'd never used it. Then you'd be out the money you spent on a product that didn't work. The products I recommend here do work.

As for silicones, there's a definite irony if you feel fine about putting in hydroxides and peroxides into your hair that will dissolve both your hair and your skin, or use searing heat from flat irons to style it, but you balk at the use of harmless silicones in a shampoo or a conditioner. I suggest the following products because they are moisturizing and don't contain sticky or stiff ingredients (see the lists of harmful ingredients under "Choosing Shampoos: What to Avoid" and "Choosing Conditioners: What to Avoid"). If you're worried about the buildup of silicones (despite the fact that if silicones build up, it simply means they weigh our hair down a little), then you can avoid shampoos and rinsing shampoos that have silicones in the ingredients. Silicones work to help a Denman-type brush comb through your curls because they are very slippery. There are a few other ingredients, however, that can provide slip as well, such as glycerin.

I don't often use the same shampoo and conditioner of a particular product line. Sometimes a company makes a great shampoo but has a bad conditioner, or it makes a wonderful conditioner yet has a harsh, drying shampoo. I tend to mix and match to get the best products.

Shampoos

Because you're applying shampoo to your scalp for only a few minutes and then rinsing it off, I'm more relaxed about shampoos. Quite a few shampoos, however—even those that say they're extremely moisturizing—contain drying ingredients. Yet there are some decent shampoos out there in basic drugstore lines, so I don't feel that it's necessary to spend more than you need to on them. Because of this, I'm listing only the shampoos that I feel are affordable. This doesn't mean there aren't some good expensive products out there. It simply means I don't see a reason to pay more for something that works the same as products that cost less. Many times, you might be paying for delicious and exotic extracts and herbs, but they won't do anything for your hair. They will hurt your wallet, though.

Although I list a few 2-in-1 shampoo plus conditioners, keep in mind that ingredients-wise, you should consider them only a slightly more moisturizing shampoo. In no way do they even come close to replacing your conditioner.

Two for One

Nearly all 2-in-1 shampoo plus conditioners are 2-in-1 because they include silicone of some type. Silicones are one of the few ingredients that don't rinse off instantly with water, so the silicone stays around to continue conditioning after the rest of your shampoo has gone down the drain. This is the "conditioning" part of the shampoo-and-conditioner.

As of the time of this writing, the products I recommend here all had gentle ingredients. I've researched the ingredients and made sure, to the best of my knowledge and research, that they don't contain any drying ingredients. There are many popular brands, some of which are known for fighting frizz and helping with dry, damaged hair, that actually have drying ingredients. I've avoided any shampoo with ingredients I know to be drying, such as sodium lauryl sulfate (see the list under "Choosing Shampoos," further on).

No-Shampoo Options

You can avoid shampooing altogether by using any of the light rinsing conditioners in place of shampoo or a cleansing conditioner such as Blended Beauty's Curl Cleansing Conditioner (see "Choosing Shampoos," further on). When you use your regular conditioner in place of your shampoo, as suggested in *Curly Girl* by Lorraine Massey, the conditioner, not a shampoo, is what grabs onto extra dirt and oils and is rinsed away. I've found that I break out if I try this with a regular conditioner, but that's because my skin's oily. If your skin is normal or dry, this might be the perfect solution, so it's worth looking into.

Recommended Shampoos

Know that products change their ingredients frequently, often without notification. Also, the same product in other countries may have different ingredients. Always check out the ingredients, even for products I recommend (there is an ingredients dictionary available at TightlyCurly.com). My favorite conditioner recently changed nearly all of its ingredients, without warning, to substances that I'm paranoid about, so I can no longer recommend it. Here are the products I do recommend:

- **Blended Beauty Soy Cream Shampoo.** This is basically a conditioner that lathers. (A biracial woman created this product line. On her Web site (blendedbeauty.com), she lists all of the ingredients in her products and explains the functions of many of the ingredients.)

- **Garnier Fructis Fortifying Shampoos.** These shampoos all have similar ingredients. All of the Garnier Fructis Fortifying Shampoos I've looked at have a large amount of silicone in them, often listed second or third after water. Silicone is a great conditioner, but if the conditioner you're leaving in your hair also has silicone, this adds up to a lot of silicone. If your hair is very dry and poufy and you feel it could use as much weight as possible, this is great. But if you want to wash out the silicone each time for a "fresh start," this might not be the best line. Conversely, the Garnier Fructis conditioners don't have enough silicone to make the comb slip through my hair easily. These might work best if you use the shampoo and the conditioner together (I tend to mix and match my shampoos and conditioners).

- **Jasön Fragrance Free Daily Shampoo.** This and the Paula's Choice shampoo have become my favorite shampoos, and both are very gentle.

- **L'Oréal Vive Pro Shampoos.** These shampoos all have similar ingredients, and as with the Garnier Fructis Fortifying Shampoos (see above), contain large amounts of silicone, which you may or may not want in a shampoo

- **Naturelle Hypo-Allergenic Fragrance Free Shampoo.** This shampoo can be found at Sally Beauty Supply stores. Though it says it's fragrance free, there are several essential oils included (such as ylang-ylang and geranium oil), that are fragrance oils, and can irritate very sensitive skin. However, the shampoo (and also the conditioner) has very little scent, so there may be only a tiny amount of these oils in them.

- **Paula's Choice.** This is the same Paula who wrote *Don't Go Shopping for Hair-Care Products without Me*. All of her products are simple, gimmick-free, no nonsense, and often multifunctional. She uses no fragrances or colors, and her products are cruelty free. On her Web site (CosmeticsCop.com), she not only lists all of the ingredients in every one of her products, but also tells you the function of each ingredient as well. I love that. In addition, her products arrive really quickly after you order them.

Medicated Shampoos

Nearly all dandruff shampoos can be harsh. Yet they go about doing what they do without too many gimmicks. To minimize the harshness, look for ones that say they are moisturizing or are for dry, damaged hair, such as Selsun Salon Moisturizing for Dry or Damaged Hair (or any of Selsun Salon's shampoos for dry, damaged, color-treated hair). For dandruff shampoos especially, it's important to use these only on your scalp to minimize their drying effect on the rest of your hair.

Good Rinsing Conditioners

Almost any conditioner for dry or damaged hair that doesn't contain any ingredients from the list to avoid would make a good rinsing conditioner. These conditioners are much lighter than the ones I recommend for leaving in (see "Good Combing Conditioners" further on). Because they're on the wimpy side, they can't do the job you need them to do when you require a robust conditioner to leave in your hair; however, they make excellent rinsers.

It's true that many more conditioners out there would be great rinsers, but the following are the cheapest, and they work just as well as those that are more expensive. So I say, why spend money when you don't have to, to do the same job?

- **Alberto VO5.** These are good, inexpensive conditioners. They all have roughly the same ingredients and all do about the same things. I choose by smell. Note that these may have too much color and fragrance for very sensitive skin, like that of a baby or a child.

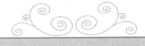

Money-Saving Tip

You can usually still use the conditioners that don't work very well and are just sitting on your bathroom shelves. The best rinsing conditioners are the ones that are more watery than the conditioners I recommend for combing. They aren't as heavy duty, but they'd be fine to rinse out your hair before you put in the real conditioner to comb your hair with, so long as they don't contain any of the ingredients you want to avoid in a hair product, listed on page 189.

Tea Therapy line of conditioners (the Calming Chamomile Tea smells really good).

Silky Experiences line of conditioners.

Moisture Milks line of conditioners.

Herbal Escapes line of conditioners.

- **Blended Beauty Curl Quenching Conditioner**
- **Nature's Gate Organics** Fruit Blend Conditioner Fortifying **Grapefruit & Wild Ginger.** This also works as a combing conditioner, but it's become my favorite rinsing conditioner. It has a soft, buttercream scent.
- **Suave Naturals** line of conditioners, so long as they say they are moisturizing. They all have roughly the same ingredients and all do about the same things. I choose by smell. Note that these may have too much color and fragrance for very sensitive skin, like that of a baby or child.
- **Trader Joe's** Essential Herbal Conditioner with Natural Fragrance.

Good Combing Conditioners

The conditioners listed here are the heavy-duty workhorses for your hair. These conditioners are strong and heavy enough to weigh down your hair but slippery enough to still allow you to comb it. Since most of these conditioners share similar ingredients, I don't feel you need to spend more than necessary on them. Because of this, I'm listing only the conditioners that I feel are affordable. Since our curly hair needs so much conditioner, there's no reason to pay more when you absolutely don't have to. This doesn't mean there aren't some good expensive products out there. It simply means I don't see any reason to pay more for something that works the same as products that cost much less. Many times, you might be paying for delicious-sounding exotic extracts and herbs, but they won't do anything for your hair.

- **Aussie Moist Conditioner.** I was stubborn and didn't try this conditioner for many years because it wasn't slippery enough back in the day when I had tried it before (I didn't know how to read labels back then). After many kind people e-mailed me to suggest I try it, I finally did. To my surprise, I loved it. I'm sure the ingredients are different now, because it combs and clumps very well. This is becoming one of my favorite combing conditioners.

- **Blended Beauty: Blended Beauty Curly Butter.** This is a good choice if you are looking for an oil-based combing conditioner that contains a larger portion of natural ingredients. It feels much like combing with a rich lotion. It's "stlippery," meaning it can get sticky if it starts to dry, but if you keep it wet, it's slippery enough to comb with. Be very gentle with your ends, however, because of the tackiness. This is a great combing conditioner if you have curls that really need to be held tightly together. However, it does tend to be greasy when it dries.

- **Giovanni 50:50 Balanced Hydrating-Calming Conditioner (for normal to dry hair).** This was another conditioner several people e-mailed and suggested I try. To my surprise, it combed well, and clumped my hair nicely.

- **Herbal Essences by Clairol.** This series of shampoos and conditioners works well. I love their fragrances. They all contain roughly the same working ingredients. The only things that change are the herbal ingredients. I go for any that say they are for dry/permed/damaged/frizzy/colored/broken hair, or that claim to be moisturizing or strengthening. After double-checking the ingredient list (see "Choosing Conditioners: The Best Ingredients to Look For," below), I usually just choose the one whose scent I like best:

  Break's Over Strengthening Conditioner (coco mango and pearls). This is my favorite scent.

  Colored/Permed/Dry/Damaged Hair Replenishing Conditioner (rosehips, vitamin E, jojoba) and shampoo. This conditioner does as good a job as the other conditioners because it has the same working ingredients. I buy it to have a variety of scents to choose from.

  Dangerously Straight Pin Straight Conditioner (honeyed pear and silk). This is also great for combing. Don't let the name throw you. It merely means it has an ingredient to help smooth your hair.

Totally Twisted Strengthening Conditioner (French lavender and jade extracts). It works as well as the other Herbal Essence conditioners with similar ingredients. I get it simply for variety, although it smells a little harsh to me.

None of Your Frizzness Strengthening Conditioner (mandarin balm and pearls). This one is also a good conditioner, similar in ingredients to the two previous conditioners. It has a nice scent.

- **Naturelle Hypo-Allergenic Fragrance Free Conditioner.** This conditioner can be found at Sally Beauty Supply stores. Though it says it's fragrance free, there are several essential oils included (such as ylang-ylang and geranium oil) that are fragrance oils and can irritate very sensitive skin. However, the conditioner (and also the shampoo) has very little scent, so there may be only a tiny amount of these oils in there. This combed and clumped my curls very well. It isn't as moisturizing as some of the other conditioners, so you can always add a bit of coconut or olive oil to your ends when they dry, or put about a teaspoon of olive oil (or other favorite emollient plant oil) in a new bottle and shake it (very hard) to mix it thoroughly before using.

- **Nexxus Hydra Sleek.** This is another great conditioner for combing. It's a bit light but perfect if you have a tough mat to get through.

- **Organix Nourishing Coconut Milk Conditioner or Shea Butter Conditioner.** These both have a nice tropical scent and comb and clump well. I was surprised these comb as well as they do, because the slippery ingredients are farther down on the label than I like to see. However, there were several slippery ingredients listed, and since it combed well, it seems there were enough of them in there to do the job.

- **Paula's Choice Smooth Finish Conditioner.** I have to say, I was really nervous to try this as a heavy-duty conditioner. It says on the bottle "All Hair Types," which I usually take to mean "Not for Hair

Like Mine." Also, my beloved silicone ingredient was listed fourth, which made me feel that if I put this in my hair, I wouldn't be able to get the comb through it. So I decided to use this as a rinsing conditioner. I was in the shower, dumped out a big handful of this conditioner to use as a rinser, and was struck by how thick it felt. So I actually put it back into the bottle, used a regular watery conditioner to rinse out, and then tried this conditioner to comb with and leave in afterward. Being nervous, I used more than I usually do. To my vast surprise, this was the smoothest combing I've ever done. If you have mats to get out of your hair, use this conditioner. It dries a little lighter than the other conditioners, however, so when you refresh your hair in the morning, you might need to use more of this product (this is what I do when I use it). This is perfect for wavier hair that doesn't need much weight or for anyone who wants a product that rinses away really easily. Despite its lightness, it's become one of my favorite combing conditioners. (See "Recommended Shampoos," above, for more about Paula.)

- **ShiKai Natural Everyday Conditioner.** This is a great conditioner. It's a bit light and barely has a scent, but it's a nice combing conditioner. It behaves much like the Paula's Choice conditioner and has also become a favorite.
- **TRESemmé.** Again, these conditioners are all basically the same, and it seems like they come out with a new one every time I look:

  Smooth & Silky for Dry or Damaged Hair. This is very thick and not as slippery as some of the other combing conditioners. If your hair is matted, this might not be the best product to use; however, it sets your curls firmly. (You could also add a little of Paula's Choice Smooth Finish Conditioner to make the combing easier.)

  Curl Moisturizing for Curly or Wavy Hair. This combed much better than the Smooth & Silky, above.

  Anti-Breakage Vitamin B-12 and Gelatin.

  Moisture Rich for Dry or Damaged Hair.

  Thermal Recovery Replenishing.

These are my personal recommendations, based on products that are currently available. I always choose the product by the first three to five ingredients listed after water (and any herbs). These are the working ingredients. Then I research to make sure there isn't anything harmful in the rest of the product. Those lovely sounding herbs and other ingredients simply make these products sound nice. Once you understand how to read a product label, you will know exactly how that product will work. (For a more up-to-date list of recommended products and ingredients, visit TightlyCurly.com. In the following sections, you'll learn how to sift through them and find the most important ingredients for your tight curls.)

How to Choose the Best Products for Your Hair

When I was a kid, I loved a certain shampoo because of the label. It showed a pretty woman, her long blond hair entwined with leaves and flowers. She looked as if she were a mermaid who had risen from the water in the middle of spring. The shampoo smelled as if the manufacturer had gathered all of those leaves and flowers, ground them up, and put them into the shampoo bottle just for me. Needless to say, when I used it, my hair did not look like the woman's on the bottle. All of the advertising, the pictures of beautiful models, and the lists of delicious herbs are irrelevant. The only thing that matters is for you to know exactly which ingredients work for you.

Once you have stopped damaging your curly hair, the most important beauty product for you is conditioner. Conditioner performs numerous duties. It's what you'll use to comb through your thick curls, it holds your curls together, and it will give them weight.

In this chapter, I suggest several excellent conditioners—as long as their ingredients stay the same as of this writing. Just in case they change or if you'd like to explore, I'll give you some guidelines for picking out good shampoos and conditioners. You'll be able to choose your products based on knowledge, not on advertising hype, pretty pictures, lists of flowers that are ground up into the product, or the inflated and misleading claims printed on the bottles.

Choosing Shampoos: What to Avoid

I tried a shampoo when I was in high school that said it could read your hair and would deposit more conditioning on the drier parts of your hair. I was so excited! Finally, my ends would start to heal, I thought. But when I rubbed the shampoo into the ends and rinsed it out, they felt as if I'd just washed them with dishwashing liquid. The shampoo didn't seem to know, after all. Because shampooing is mostly for the scalp, it's not crucial to get the perfect one. Choose the shampoo according to what your scalp needs and the conditioner based on what your hair needs. It isn't necessary to buy an expensive shampoo, either. Cheap shampoos will do just fine. I often choose by smell, as long as there isn't anything on the list of ingredients to avoid (see the harmful substances detailed in "Choosing Conditioners: What to Avoid," as well as those in the following list).

- Sodium lauryl sulfate is drying. (Sodium *laureth* sulfate is fine. It's gentle.)
- Ammonium xylenesulfate is a lacquer solvent and can be very drying.
- TEA-laurylsulfate is drying and might cause skin irritation.
- TEA-dodecylbenzene is drying.
- TEA-dodecylbenzenesulfonate can strip color from your hair, as well as dry it out.
- Alkyl sodium sulfate is drying and might cause skin irritation.
- Sodium dodecylbenzenesulfonate is often found in dishwashing liquids because it is very strong and very cheap. It can cause skin irritation.
- Sodium coco-sulfate is basically the same thing as sodium lauryl sulfate. This means it's a harsh cleanser.
- Alkyl benzene sulfonate is harsh, irritating, and drying. It's known for being a good defatter, which means it's good at stripping oils from surfaces.
- Sodium C14-16 olefin sulfonate is drying and can cause skin irritation.

Choosing Conditioners: The Best Ingredients to Look For

The best conditioners are those that make it easier to comb tight curls and help set them and give them weight (when curls have weight, they tend to stay clumped better, and have more motion). The three most important ingredient types you should look for (after water—keep in mind that water still functions the same, even when it's "tea water," as Paula Begoun calls water with lots of herbs seeped in it) and in this order are: weight ingredients, slip ingredients, and moisturizing ingredients.

Weight Ingredients

These are the ingredients that keep your curls clumped together and your hair hanging more or less vertically, instead of rising horizontally in rain or humidity (if you don't want them to become horizontal, that is). Ingredients classified as thickeners, fatty alcohols, fatty acids, many quaternary ammonium compounds (some of these ingredients function to give products more slip in addition to weight), lubricants, and emollients and antistatic ingredients will function in this way. Stearyl alcohol is my favorite, with cetyl alcohol and cetearyl alcohol close seconds (these aren't the same as isopropyl alcohol, or ethanol —which is rubbing alcohol, also known as SD alcohol, or ethyl alcohol). Ingredients such as behentrimonium chloride, quaternarium 18, stearalkonium chloride, and cetrimonium chloride are fine, too. These ingredients are nongreasy lubricants and thickeners, so they make the product, and thus your hair when you comb it, nice and slippery. When they dry, they help give your curls some weight and keep it moist without oiliness, stickiness, or crunchiness.

Slip Ingredients

These are ingredients that make it possible to get the Denman-type brush through your hair with minimal force and therefore minimal damage. Silicones (such as dimethicone or cyclomethicone) work wonders in helping the brush glide through your hair. My favorite slippery ingredients are silicones, such as cyclopentasiloxane, which is a silicone that evaporates from your hair once it dries. Glycerin also works well to create slip, and much to my surprise, stearamidopropyl dimethylamine also seems to add slip to a product. These substances work best if they are listed as the second or third ingredient (not counting water), after the weight ingredient. Though I must say I've been surprised to find conditioners with their slip ingredients listed fourth or even fifth after the weight ingredients, and they are still slippery enough for combing. This is most likely because all of the weight ingredients listed were in smaller portions each. So perhaps all of them combined equaled the proportion of a single weight ingredient listed in other products. As long as the slip ingredient is listed immediately after the weight ingredients (and not down by the fragrances, colors, or preservatives) the product has a chance at being slippery enough to comb with.

Conditioners don't seem to have enough weight if the slippery ingredient is first, directly after water. This is because most of the slip ingredients tend to evaporate when they dry. Because ingredients are listed in the order of their proportions, it means that when the slip ingredient is listed after water, most of the product will evaporate by the time your hair dries. This leaves your curls free to un-clump and expand. I like my curls to be well defined, so I tend to go for products that show off their texture and keep them together. If the weight ingredient is listed right after water (or the tea water, depending on the conditioner) as the second ingredient, it's this ingredient that remains behind and makes sure your hair stays calm and collected. You still want to see your slip ingredient high up on the list, however, because you need plenty of it for your Denman-type brush to glide through your curls with minimal friction.

Moisturizing Ingredients

These help keep your curls glossy and moisturized. I don't like to see them listed before weight or slip ingredients because in this high of a percentage, they tend to make the product really greasy and the conditioner might not give your hair enough weight (or slip for the comb to get through). But I do like to see them as soon after the weight and slip ingredients as possible. Great moisturizing ingredients are often oils or butters, such as olive oil, avocado oil, meadowfoam seed oil, coconut oil, shea butter, jojoba oil, palm oil, and sunflower oil.

An excellent oil to smooth on the ends of your hair at night before putting it up is coconut oil. A study conducted by the *Journal of Cosmetic Science* showed that this oil can penetrate the hair shaft and may help increase its strength (but, of course, nothing can repair damaged hair). The same study found that mineral oil didn't penetrate the hair much at all. Most of the natural oils are highly moisturizing, however, and I tend to simply use olive oil occasionally on my ends in winter.

Why Silicones?

I know some of you might believe that silicone-based products are bad for your hair. This simply isn't true. I've been using them heavily for years, and my hair looks better than it has for most of my life. Don't miss out on something that could genuinely help you, based on secondhand information. When you read warnings about silicone-based products, you must always ask yourself, Where did the source get his or her information?

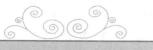

Not All Silicones Are Alike

Although silicones generally aren't water soluble, some silicones, such as cyclomethicone and cyclopentasiloxane, do evaporate. This means that while your hair is wet, they help make it slippery enough to comb. And by the time your hair dries, they're gone.

At a picnic a few years ago, a family member asked me about my favorite brand of conditioner, and a close family friend overheard my answer. She came running up to us, clutching her wig so that it wouldn't fall off, to say that I was wrong, totally wrong. She knew the perfect product to use and insisted vehemently that her conditioner worked far better than mine did. She was really convincing, too—however, I'd seen the peach fuzz beneath her wig when one of her kids snatched it from her head and ran off with it. What I'm saying is that anyone can insist that she has the answers for you. But look at the source, find out where the person's information came from, and look at what's really going on beneath the surface. (Are they telling you this to justify selling you expensive products? Are they misrepresenting studies to slant these in their favor?) Don't believe something just because it's said to you with authority or because you've heard it so often, you assume it must be true.

Whenever people give me hair-care advice, unless they can tell me which studies they're using to support what they're saying, I always look at their hair. Do they have hair like mine, so that I know they understand my issues? Is their hair long and healthy? If it's short because it's breaking off or they can't grow it because it's damaged, I tend not to listen. (I know, I'm paranoid. But I'm a paranoid with long hair.) What *objective scientific* studies can they show me? Be aware that many companies pay for the very studies that "prove" their products work.

Just because something is human-made doesn't make it bad. Think of all the vaccines and the medicines that are people-made and that save lives every day. And, conversely, just because something is natural doesn't mean it's automatically good for you or will work for you. Poison oak, poison ivy, stinging nettle, and hemlock are all natural ingredients, but I try to avoid them whenever I can.

A great book to read is *Don't Go Shopping for Hair-Care Products without Me* by Paula Begoun. She cuts through all of the advertising misinformation. She's also read the actual scientific studies done on the ingredients and their effects on hair and even tells you exactly where her information comes from. Begoun wrote, "Silicone not only provides temporary renewed smoothness to the hair, but also is the subject of an enormous amount of research (that fills several folders in my office) demonstrating its extraordinary safety . . . consider it your dry, coarse, frizzy, damaged, brittle, over styled, wiry, rough, hard-to-comb hair's best friend."

There are many myths regarding why silicones are bad for hair. I read about one concern that hair can't "breathe" if it's coated in silicone. As you'll remember from chapter 2, however, hair isn't alive, and therefore it isn't doing any breathing of any kind. Yet too much of any heavy product, including silicones and natural oils, can build up and clog the pores on your scalp. So it's best not to let any products pile up on your scalp.

There's also a myth that silicone coats hair and prevents moisture from getting through. According to *The Beauty Brains* Web site at TheBeauty Brains.com, there is no research to support this belief. Silicone, in fact, surrounds each strand of hair in a moisturizing glove, actually protecting it from moisture loss.

Although many silicones evaporate from hair, the ones that remain may potentially build up on hair. From my research, it sounds like the biggest downside to silicones when they build up is that they can weigh your hair down. If you think about it, isn't that exactly what you need them to do? The whole reason I leave conditioners in my hair is to give my hair weight and to keep it clumped together and moisturized, since I usually like my curls defined. Even after I walk in the rain for hours, my hair is still calm, and my curls are still defined. On the other hand, this advice that silicones are bad and build up makes sense if you have straighter hair that's easily flattened. Then, yes, you should avoid them. But for those of us with very curly hair, silicones are a glorious thing.

Choosing Conditioners: What to Avoid

On any bottle of product you are looking at, there will be a listing of numerous other ingredients after the recommended ones (see earlier in this chapter), and it's good to look over these as well. Although any ingredients named at the beginning of the list make up the bulk of the product, the function of the product can change if one of the following ingredients is lurking in the list. Know that any ingredients listed near the bottom, especially anything after the fragrance, will be present in very small amounts. This means you really only need to scan the list to make sure there's nothing undesirable in the product.

Sticky or Crunchy

Avoid sticky or holding ingredients that are sometimes put in conditioners. These sometimes appear in products for "frizzy" hair, and they are used to keep the hairs stuck together. This isn't good for your curls. You're already using the conditioner itself to give your curls weight and keep them together, without stiffness or stickiness. Products with sticky or holding ingredients tend to keep your comb from gliding through your hair and will build up in your hair. Avoid products with ingredients that have names with copolyol anything, acrylate anything, vinyl anything, or PVP anything. It was these ingredients that made my hair feel like the back of a sticky note.

Rubbing Alcohol

Avoid products with grain or rubbing alcohol in them, such as SD alcohol 40, isopropyl alcohol, ethanol, or ethyl alcohol, because these tend to be drying to your hair.

Salt

This might just be my paranoia talking, but some conditioners out there have salt up near the top of the ingredient list. Salt is often used as an inexpensive thickening ingredient. Because I'm leaving conditioner in my hair, however, and salt is corrosive, I'm going to avoid anything with sodium chloride, sodium bicarbonate (baking soda), or potassium chloride.

How to Pick Your Own Conditioners

Before you try to read the ingredient list of every single bottle of conditioner in the store, or worse, simply believe what the advertising promises and buy that product, it's best to start with a plan. This section simplifies your search into something doable.

Narrowing It Down

First, head for any conditioner that indicates it was made for any type of dry or damaged hair, even though your hair should no longer be damaged after you follow the tips in this book for a while. Products geared toward dry or damaged hair have basically the same ingredients, which tend to be more conditioning. Specific problems are used as a marketing technique. If you have color-treated hair and are concerned about it, you'll be more likely to grab a bottle of conditioner that says it's for color-treated hair, rather than one for permed hair, even though the ingredients in both bottles might be nearly identical. We all like to feel that a product was designed only for us, and the advertisers know it. Without reading the back of the bottle, there's no way to know what you're getting.

Aim for conditioners for the most dire-sounding hair problems possible. These are more likely to have the most conditioning ingredients. Anything geared toward permed, colored, damaged, dry, broken, relaxed, bleached, depressed, or very curly hair is best to begin with. Even if your hair doesn't have any of these problems, the goal is to find the most conditioning product out there. These words are flags signaling you that a certain product might be a good candidate to look at.

Check the Labels

Once you have a potential product in hand, quickly scan the label. Most conditioners that are both slippery enough to help you comb your hair and heavy enough to weigh your curls have the big three listed as their first three ingredients after water (or any variation of water plus herbs):

1. A weight ingredient like stearyl alcohol, cetyl alcohol, or cetearyl alcohol
2. The all-important slip ingredient like cyclomethicone, glycerin, or cyclopentasiloxane
3. Emollient ingredients such as shea butter, jojoba, coconut oil, or olive oil (these are nice to have in there, but the first two types of ingredients are the most crucial)

If those first two ingredients aren't there, put the conditioner bottle down and keep looking. No matter what else is in the product, it won't be able to do its job without those ingredients, so the rest of the list is irrelevant. This will save you so much time when scanning labels. You will now be able to go through the conditioner aisle and very quickly assess whether a bottle is even worth your reading through the entire list. If those three ingredients are present, that takes care of the good stuff. The conditioner will work if those three ingredients are there. It's that simple. The only thing you have to check now is to make sure the manufacturer didn't slip in something that would impede the first three ingredients from working.

Next, check to see whether any unwanted ingredients are listed. Bad ingredients are anything sticky, such as PVP anything (such as PVP/VA copolymer), copolymer anything (for example, acrylamide copolymer), acrylate anything (such as acrylamide or acrylate copolymer), vinyl anything (like vinyl acetate or polyvinyl acetate), and rubbing alcohol–type ingredients (such as isopropyl alcohol, ethyl alcohol, and SD alcohol 40).

It sounds like a lot to look for, but the ingredients you want to avoid all have a similar sound to them. Once you're familiar with the gist of their names, even though you won't remember a specific name, you'll recognize the dreaded sound of an "acrylate copolymer," for example. Or something plastic-sounding like "vinyl." A small chill will go down your back when you read one of these ingredients listed on a label.

Any extra bells and whistles are nice but not necessary, such as vitamin E (tocopherol), proteins, panthenols, or exotic-sounding oils that are most likely there for show. It's great to have even more plant oils in the product. Just keep in mind that if you have your first three ingredient types after water (weight, slip, and moisturizing), these will be doing the bulk of the work. They will be like the big Clydesdale horses pulling the wagon. The other ingredients are more like the little yipping puppies running alongside.

Never Go For . . .

- **Leave-ins.** Never go for a product that calls itself a leave-in conditioner. These come in two basic flavors: One type is little more than water. It is meant to be put in limp hair and not weigh it down. This is the opposite of what we need. Our hair won't even notice it's in there. The second type tends to have greasy and/or sticky ingredients that can build up and become difficult to rinse out. The ingredients you need, you can find in conditioners.

- **Volumizers.** Don't try conditioners marketed for thin, limp hair or ones that say they increase volume. Again, these are not for us and produce the opposite effect of what we are trying to do. Volumizing products usually work by making the hair sticky. The last thing you need is sticky hair.

- **Other Tricky Ingredients.** With these, I'm not saying don't go for them. Some ingredients, like glycerin, do a really good job when you know what their function should be. It's just that some of these products are used in misleading ways, so you need to be cautious when you see them.

Glycerin. When I was still trying to find the perfect product that could weigh my hair down and keep my curls clumped without being crunchy, I once bought something marketed specifically for just that: to help weigh down curls and keep them from frizzing. It even had a picture of a mixed-ethnicity woman with long curls on it. I was so happy to see her on that bottle! I bought it immediately and slathered it into my hair. It worked for the first hour I had it in—while it was still wet, that is. Unfortunately, as it began to dry, my curls drew back up again and then puffed apart like I'd put nothing on them. It turned out that the main ingredient was glycerin.

Glycerin feels nice and slippery when it's applied; however, it dries up quickly, and then it's gone like dew in the afternoon. It's best to regard any product with this ingredient as slippery water. It's great for combing out our hair because it's so slippery. But when it dries, it's gone. Because of this, we need more robust conditioning ingredients in our products. We need them to take over once the glycerin dries up and disappears.

Vaseline (petroleum jelly). It can be a bit greasy and thick, and it's known for being difficult to rinse off with water. A conditioner with this near the top of the ingredient list might be too thick to use to comb your hair with. In small amounts, however (meaning that you'll find it far down on the ingredient list), it should be okay.

Frizz-tamers. The majority of frizz-tamers are composed of silicone-like ingredients. Silicones are wonderful for combing and moisturizing our hair, but they work by coating your hair with a slippery substance. You could use an entire bottle in your hair, and it wouldn't define your curls. These products don't work. Ignore the before-and-after photos. They had a team of hairdressers first rat the model's hair to look awful. Then the hairdressers washed and set her hair to look smooth. What works is the technique, not the product. Products only enhance what you are doing. Believe me, I bought so many bottles of frizz-tamers, and when I continued to look like the model in the before photos, it made me feel as if my hair fell outside the orbit of help.

Curl enhancers. Be cautious if something says it's for emphasizing or creating curls or to tame frizz. These sometimes have sticky, gel-like ingredients in them to keep hair stuck together. Just double-check to make sure they don't have acrylates, PVP, copolyol anything, or vinyl anything. These products just might be extra conditioning, however, so they can be worth a look.

Curl flatteners. I know it seems like a contradiction, but even though you want to emphasize your curls, conditioners that say they're for straightening curls can be okay, too. Many of them work by laying on some extra conditioning and smoothing ingredients, like silicones. Again, check for sticky ingredients.

Conditioning henna. Sometimes you'll see henna advertised to help with shine. You buy it and put it on, and it's supposed to add lots of gloss. First, I'll say that the only way to have healthy, glossy hair is to learn how to treat it and stop damaging it. Second, henna can build up in your hair and dry it out. Third, I once tried a colorless henna treatment to try to get some shine in my hair, back in the days when I was looking for a magic product. I got a kit that included a bag of ground henna. Following the directions, I mixed it with water and then applied it to my hair. I let it sit, then, after a certain amount of time, I rinsed it off. For most people this would have been fine. For my hair, nothing is that simple.

I rinsed and rinsed and rinsed. The ground herb stuck fast between every strand of hair. When I finally thought I'd gotten it all out, I combed my hair. I combed out piles of that ground henna. When my hair dried, I discovered that the henna had been embedded into my hair because I'd combed it. I'd shake my head, and henna would rain down to settle on my shoulders in attractive beige flakes. It took weeks to get it out of my hair.

The "Natural" Myth

I love the thought of using natural products. During the three decades when I searched for answers for my hair, a good portion of my quest consisted of trying natural products. When I read the labels listing exotic herbs and flowers, I imagined someone going out to a lovely summer meadow, picking a basket of fragrant flowers and herbs, and then preparing sweetly scented products with them.

Yet no matter how much a bottle containing natural ingredients cost me, it never helped my damaged hair. I know I keep saying it, but the only thing that helps our hair is to stop damaging it and to treat it like curly hair. No product in the world can take the place of that. As Paula Begoun said in *Don't Go Shopping for Hair Care Products without Me*, "All of the plants and vitamins in the world can't bring a dead leaf back to life, or put fallen petals back on a rose, and they can't change the very dead hair on your head."

Natural products are often expensive, and it's best to know the truth before you spend lots of money on them so you can make an informed decision and buy them for the right reasons. There is evidence, however, that herbs, vitamins, and certain oils have various benefits for your skin and body. This is because your skin and body are living things and have the ability to incorporate nutrients into living tissue. Hair is dead, though, and herbs are simply washed down the drain when you rinse your hair with them, no matter how much they cost you. If you absolutely love using natural products, you could use one of the cheaper, functional workhorse products for combing (because you need to use lots to do so) and then use a favorite natural product for rinsing and to smooth your hair in the morning.

For a dictionary of the ingredients contained in hair-care products (and whether they hurt or help), go to TightlyCurly.com.

The Best Hair Tools for Your Curls

Once you have all the pieces of the puzzle on how to take care of your curls, your hair suddenly becomes relatively simple. If you are using even one of the wrong tools, however, you may still be left with broken, tangled hair that hurts to comb, or you end up having to cut out a barrette. Here are some of the tools that have made caring for my curls so much easier.

Your Brush

The most important styling tool will be your brush. This is what builds your curls. The right brush will actually cut down on the damage caused by combing hair wet. I have used the terms *brush* and *comb* interchangeably in the book, because the combing is being done by a particular style of brush. This is the Denman brush or a Denman-style brush. They are usually found in salon stores, and they cost a bit more than a regular brush, but they are worth the price. These are good, sturdy brushes that will not fall apart when combing thick hair; they have "give" in their bases, so they will be gentle on your hair. The best Denman-type brush is a styling brush with a rubber base and seven to nine rows of rounded nylon teeth. Every row has about twenty-two teeth each. They come in different colors but are most often found with a black or white handle and a red rubber base. The rubber base has a great deal of give, so the

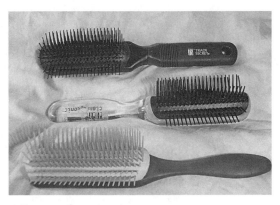

A Denman-type brush.

give comes from your brush and not from your vulnerable hair. The nylon teeth are smooth and rounded. Never get a brush that has teeth with balls on the ends, because your hair will tangle on every one of them.

When I was searching for a way to comb my hair, I used to buy cheap drugstore brushes. If the brushes didn't fall apart the moment I tried to tug them though my curls, they fell apart within a few uses. Our hair is heavy-duty hair. It needs a good, giving, but strong brush. I think it's best to try out a Denman first, so you can see what it does and how well it holds up to your curls. Then you can branch out and try other brushes that work the same as a Denman.

When you first use this brush, brush with it gently. Be careful not to accidentally smack your head with it when your hair is wet. And keep in mind that *any* brush will damage your hair if used roughly.

As mentioned, you can find Denman brushes at beauty supply stores and at www.DenmanBrush.com. I use the D4 Classic Styling brush with nine rows of nylon pins, but the D3 is fine too (it's a bit smaller, with seven rows of pins).

Holding-Your-Hair Tools

The best items to use for your hair are as simple as possible. Look for things that seem almost primitive. The fewer grooves, hinges, and working parts, the fewer places your curls can catch on and tangle. Sometimes, when I shop for a new item, I run it lightly over my hair. If it tangles, I don't buy it. It's better for you to discover that it will knot up in your hair before you've spent the money on it than to find out later. Also, check the teeth or any surface that will be in contact with your hair, and make sure there are no rough edges, especially those on the inside of the plastic tortoiseshell pins. If there's a rough spot in the seam, it will tear at your hair when it is put in and taken out.

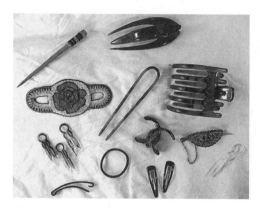

The best hair accessories.

Most of the hair tools in the photo above can be found at any drugstore and at www.Scunci.com. The best pins to hold up thick curls are available at some beauty supply stores and at www.GoodHairDays.com or Scunci.

Rubber Bands

Never use plain rubber bands, such as the kind taken off a newspaper. You will be cutting the band and chunks of your hair out every time you try to remove it. Always use the kind of band that is meant for hair, one covered in nylon or a thin fabric. It's best to put the band for a ponytail on loosely. Your curls will hold the band in your hair. Wrapping a band around your hair in a stranglehold will break your hair from the stress of being too tight. For a low, loose tail, a smaller band wrapped once is all right, or use a larger band doubled so that it just holds your hair back. Make sure your hair has breathing room inside the band.

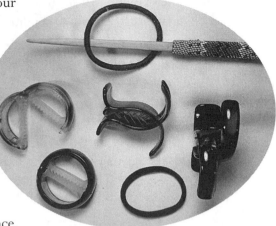

Some of the different types of clips you can use.

For a higher, firmer tail, you can use a clip with handles that squeeze open; then put your curls in it and close it firmly in place. Try to use a clip that has larger teeth but fewer of them. The best clip that I've found for a high pony-tail has only three prongs, which keeps the tail close to my head. Using a clip instead of a band saves wear and tear on your hair. Wrapping a band repeatedly in your hair while pulling very long curls through, over and over, to tighten it will produce too much stress on both hair and scalp, with no relief, because the severe band holds tight all day.

Gels

I almost never use gel. Leaving conditioner in my hair does everything I need. Even so, I have a low hairline, so there are several inches of hair to hang over my eyes. My curls are thick and seem happiest when they're draped over my face, so I need something strong to hold them back— sort of like a dam. I consider this product to be more of a spot-welding service and apply it only in the area where I need help, and only for special occasions. That's why I go for the strength of a spiking gel or paste. Know that a little product does go a long way, and it can make the spot you put it in as hard as papier-mâché. If this happens, you can simply go over it with water and dab it with a paper towel to absorb the excess.

On the very rare occasions when I might use gel, I don't worry too much about the ingredients in it. I use gel only to hold my hair in place in certain spots, so sticky ingredients on the ingredients list are expected.

I've found that the best ones to keep my curls off my face are spiking gels and pastes. Because conditioner keeps my curls well formed, I need the gel only for the specific purpose of holding back my front hair. I look for a holding paste that sounds somewhat conditioning, but I know what its purpose is, and most of the pastes seem to fulfill it. To be honest, with these products, I go with whatever smells good since I use it so rarely, and only at a small area of my hairline.

When I was a child, I often hid in the bathroom and mixed conditioners together into concoctions. Then I stashed them in tiny containers under the sink and in the cabinets. I was certain that I was hot on the trail of

Take Away Tips

- Shampoo is for your scalp; conditioner is for your hair.
- Look for conditioners that have weight ingredients first, slip second, and moisturizing ingredients that appear before the fragrance is listed.
- Silicone is your curly hair's friend.
- Avoid sticky ingredients such as copoly anything, acrylate anything, vinyl anything, or PVP anything.
- Avoid rubbing-type alcohol in conditioners, such as isopropyl, ethyl, or SD alcohol.
- Natural ingredients can't heal your hair. They're natural, not magic.
- Some products are advertised as being natural, when in fact they use the same working ingredients as drugstore brands. These companies simply charge you more.
- Not everything natural is good, and not everything made by people is bad.
- Look for hair tools that are as simple as possible.
- The best brush for our hair is a Denman (or Denman-type) brush.

inventing a new substance. I felt that when the products I'd combined had dried, they would form some amazing substance never before seen, and I'd be the only person who could produce it. I never did find out whether I'd made any new substance. My containers kept mysteriously disappearing.

After all this time, at least now I know what the substances inside the conditioners actually are and what they can and can't do.

Chapter Twelve

Chemically Altering Your Hair
The Truth behind Coloring, Perming, and Relaxing

As I have a tendency to mention whenever I have a chance, when I was seventeen, I accidentally dissolved my hair with a relaxer. I had no idea what the chemicals would do when I applied them or what reactions would take place when these chemicals were used. At the time, I only cared that they did what I'd bought them to do. I mistook familiarity for safety, and I lost an entire head of hair because I didn't know any better. If you are equipped with a basic understanding of what actually happens to your hair when you apply chemicals, *you* can make informed choices on behalf of your hair.

There are two ways you can permanently alter your hair with chemicals (well, at least until it grows out again): coloring it and altering its texture. This chapter covers what happens to your hair, on a molecular level, when hair-coloring and texture-altering chemicals are applied to your curls. To grasp how extreme the damage can be, you need to understand how these chemicals change the basic structure of your hair, as well as be aware of the aftereffects of this change. You need to know what happens inside the black box, between the time you put chemicals on your hair and the time you rinse them out again.

What Happens When You Change the Color of Your Hair?

The color of your hair is produced by melanin pigments scattered like Easter eggs through the cortex of your hair shafts. Two pigments in your hair give it its color: eumelanin and phaeomelanin. Eumelanin is the main pigment in darker hair. It gives your hair a range of shades from red-brown to black. Phaeomelanin is the main pigment in lighter hair colors. It gives hair a light yellow or red color. The exact shade of your hair depends on the mixture of pigments that are present. If there aren't any pigment granules in the cortex, it looks yellowish-white at the roots. This is because keratin itself is slightly yellow and is the only thing contributing to the hair color. Gray hair isn't actually gray; it merely looks that way. It's actually a mixture of white and colored hairs that appear gray when seen together.

There are four basic ways to alter the color of your hair: temporary, semipermanent and permanent color, and lightening. The effects these have on your hair range from relatively harmless to damaging.

Temporary Coloring

Temporary hair color lasts only until the next time you wash your hair. This process does not contain any peroxides. Temporary color works by coating your cuticles with a pigment composed of large molecules. This forms a film or a stain on your hair. The coloring is slightly acidic, so when the stain is applied, the cuticles snap shut in response to this acidic environment. Keeping the cuticles tightly shut ensures that the large molecules of the stain can't get inside, to the cortex. The color molecules sit on the cuticle with nothing to anchor them, like sticky jellybeans on a fence. They wash away easily with the next shampooing. Due to the coating on your hair (as well as any potentially damaging ingredients that may be in the formula), temporary hair coloring may be drying to your hair.

Semipermanent Color

Semipermanent treatments can last from six to twelve weeks. These don't use any peroxides to work but are slightly alkaline. Applying a semipermanent color causes your hair shaft to swell slightly in response to the alkaline environment, and this causes the cuticles to open slightly, like millions of drawbridges. The color molecules used are small, so they pass easily inside the raised cuticles. A slightly neutral-to-acidic rinse is applied to close the cuticles again, trapping the color molecules between the shingles. When your hair is washed, the cuticles open slightly. This allows the tiny dye molecules to slip out. Over time and with repeated washings, these molecules are washed away. Because of this, semipermanent colors can't change the color of your hair, only stain it. Depending on how alkaline the formula is, semipermanent hair coloring may cause minor damage to your cuticles, as well as cause some dryness to your hair.

Permanent Dyes

Permanent dyes are alkaline, often using a highly basic compound such as ammonium hydroxide, or ethanolamine, to cause the hair shaft to swell and open the cuticles. The pH needed in order for the dye to work is very high (about 10 to 11) enough to cause damage to your hair with this pH alone. (I discuss what exactly pH means later on in this chapter, under "About the pH Used in Perms and Relaxers.") The coloring molecules of permanent dyes start out innocently enough: tiny and colorless. Immediately before the dye is applied to your hair, it's mixed with hydrogen peroxide to activate the color. Because of the small size of the dye molecules, they easily pass between the scales of the opened cuticles, into the cortex. The added hydrogen peroxide reacts with these molecules, making them expand and turn colored. These swollen molecules are now too plump to pass back through the cuticle, so they remain permanently lodged in place. No matter how moisturizing or natural the box of dye tells you that it is, the high alkalinity needed to swell your hair in order to open your cuticles for the dye to work (not to mention the hydrogen peroxide) will damage your hair.

Lightening Your Hair

Hair is usually lightened with hydrogen peroxide, because it reacts with the melanin pigments in the cortex. A highly alkaline solution (with a pH of 10 to 11), often made with ammonia, is first applied to your hair. This solution opens your cuticles and prompts the hydrogen peroxide to do its thing and to react faster with the melanin pigments. When the melanin grains react with the hydrogen peroxide, they turn colorless, like little ghosts. Once altered, the ghostly melanin granules are dissolved in the alkaline environment and are rinsed from the hair, leaving little empty spots in the cortex.

Peroxide reacts differently with the eumelanin than with the phaeomelanin pigments in your hair. Peroxide lightens the darker eumelanin faster than it does the lighter-colored phaeomelanin. Because both are present in varying amounts in your hair, the darker eumelanin is quickly changed to a colorless substance that's rinsed away. This exposes the more stubborn red- or yellow-colored phaeomelanin molecules that were previously hidden behind the darker eumelanin pigments. If a more radical change of color is desired, a two-step process is performed. This involves stripping all of the natural color from your hair with a strong hydrogen peroxide solution. The strong solution removes both the eumelanin and the phaeomelanin from your hair and then replaces them with a new color. According to hair and skin expert Dr. John Gray, bleaching destroys the protein, keratin, that makes up your hair. As described in chapter 2, keratin is the very foundation of the hair's structure. The damage from this process can be severe, and can turn previously soft hair into brittle hay.

The Aftereffects of Lightening

Anything that chemically alters your hair will cause damage. Lightening your hair with peroxides, especially the powerful ones that are needed to drastically lighten your hair by several shades, can rupture disulfide bonds that hold the fiber of your hair together. After a bout of lightening, your cuticles become weakened. When they're weakened, even simple things like combing can easily tear them off. Bleached hair is more porous than virgin hair, so it swells more when wet. Unfortunately, being wet also makes it weaker, so now it's like a worn paper towel (see chapter 2).

Bleaching your hair will result in it becoming dry and brittle and more prone to tangling. It will also become rougher to the touch. The more drastically your hair is bleached, the rougher it will feel. This means your cuticles are no longer lying flat. These raised cuticles are soon torn off and eroded away through regular combing, leaving the cortex exposed. Once exposed, the cortex quickly unravels. In electron micrograph photos, it looks like the cortexes have exploded.

About the pH Used in Perms and Relaxers

Perms and relaxers use a strong pH to do their work. The term *pH* describes the degree of acidity or alkalinity a substance has. As a reference: lemon juice is an acidic 2, tomato juice is 4, skin is slightly acidic between 5 and 6, pure water is neutral at 7, household ammonia is alkaline at 11.5, bleach is 12.5, and oven cleaners and drain cleaners are highly alkaline, with a pH of about 13.5. Because they're so alkaline, oven and drain cleaners eat rapidly through oils, fats, aluminum, skin, and hair. The chemicals that are used to take curls out of your hair are also highly alkaline. They're between pH 9 and all the way up to relaxers that top out at 14. Yup, that relaxer's pH is as high as the pH in drain cleaners. Chemicals that are used to alter your hair *do not* mess around.

An Overview of the Processes

When the alkaline chemicals are placed on your hair, your hair begins to swell. As each hair swells, its cuticles lift like scales stuck onto an expanding balloon. When your cuticles lift, the cortex is exposed. There's nothing it can do to shield itself once its protective covering is gone. The doors are now open for the chemicals to enter the heart of your hair. Once inside, they break all of your hydrogen bonds and swarm the disulfide scaffolding that holds your hair together. As the chemicals react with the disulfide links, they break these, too, undoing the fastenings that hold your hair together. Your hair softens and bloats further because those reinforcing girders are breaking. Your hair becomes putty, and now that it's softened and defenseless, it can be molded into a new shape.

In this plastic state, your hair is combed to stretch out its curls. The broken disulfide links are repositioned to conform in this new shape. When your hair is neutralized, the disulfide bonds are set with new partners in their new positions. Neutralizing rinses your hair in an acidic solution (with a pH of 3 to 4), which returns your hair to its regular pH and hardens it. This new shape is locked in when the bonds re-form. Once re-formed, the bonds can't return to their previous positions.

Two basic types of chemicals are used to permanently remove the curls from curly hair. They perform different chemical changes in your hair and cause various levels of damage. Although the terms are commonly used interchangeably, *straightening* and *relaxing* refer to different products that leave very different hair fibers in their wake. Depending on which chemicals are used in this process, two different fates occur to the broken bonds when they re-form.

Chemically Removing Your Curls

In chapter 2, I mentioned the tenacious disulfide bonds that hold your hair together and give it shape. These bonds reinforce the curl of your hair up and down the length of every strand, millions of times over. They're embedded in the countless alpha helices that make up the fiber of your hair. Most of your hair's strength comes from these links. And it's these bonds that must be broken for your hair to be chemically straightened. Because these bonds are ferociously strong, it takes brutal chemicals to break them.

What Happens When You Straighten Your Hair?

A straightener uses thioglycolate. This is the same active ingredient that people with straight hair use when they get perms to curl their hair. Thioglycolate is often sold in stores for Jheri curls. These products containing thioglycolate have a pH of around 8.5 to 9.6.

When the thioglycolate product is placed on your hair, the alkaline pH causes your hair shaft to swell. The swelling forces cuticles apart in the same way that dried paint would crack on an expanding balloon. When the protective cuticles have been opened, the chemicals begin to work on the structure of the cortex. The chemicals break all of the hydrogen bonds. They break apart the sulfur bridges by inserting a hydrogen atom between

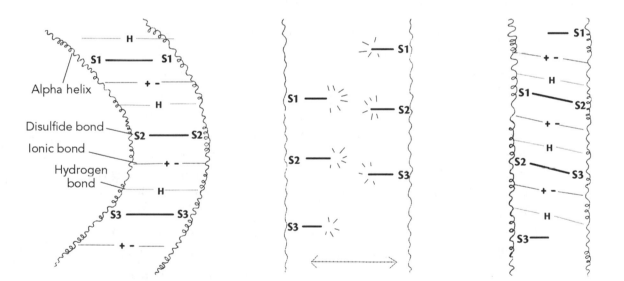

What happens when you straighten your hair.

Before straightening:	During straightening:	After straightening:
All bonds are present.	In the alkaline environment all H and ionic bonds are broken, and most disulfide bonds are broken. Hair swells and softens and can be formed into its new position.	Bonds are realigned with different partners and re-formed. Not all bonds form again.

them. With the hair's support system broken, the hair continues to swell and soften. It's now time to set it in its new position, whether curlier or straighter.

As your hair is shaped, either on rods or combed straight, the broken sulfur links slide into new positions. Once your hair is in its new shape, it's neutralized. This locks the bonds back together in their new positions. To get really technical, during neutralization, oxygen is introduced to the hair in the form of a peroxide. The oxygen from the peroxide attracts the hydrogen back out from between the sulfide bridges so they can re-link. When the sulfur bridges form again, they form with new partners in new positions. Because most of the sulfur bonds link back together again, only with new partners, your hair retains its elasticity and most of its strength.

What Happens When You Relax Your Hair?

Relaxer refers to any product that has a hydroxide as its active ingredient, such as sodium hydroxide, calcium hydroxide, potassium hydroxide, lithium hydroxide, or guanidine hydroxide. The pH of these chemicals is much higher than in thioglycolate perms, between 10 and 14. Sodium hydroxide is also known as "soda lye," the same lye that's used in oven cleaners and drain cleaners. Manufacturers distance themselves from this stigma by using another type of hydroxide and calling their products "no-lye," but it's about semantics more than substance. Chemically, they're very similar to each other, and they all do the same thing to your hair that lye does.

When the hydroxides are applied, their high pH causes your hair to swell, as it does with thioglycolate, forcing the cuticles apart and exposing the cortex. The hydroxides in relaxers, though, have a scarier pH and break down all of the hydrogen bonds and most of the sulfide bonds. Now that the structural support for your hair fibers is broken, your hair swells considerably. Each hair can swell up to three times its original size, much like pasta when it's cooked. And like cooked pasta, your hair becomes rubbery. In this state, it can be shaped. Relaxers are usually thick, to make it easier to smooth back tight curls and hold them in the new position.

Inside each hair, the broken sulfurs are moved into new positions. Once the sulfurs are in the new positions, your hair is rinsed and neutralized. This is much like shaping the cooked pasta and setting it out to dry again. When it's dry, the new shape is set.

Unfortunately, the relaxing process removes one of the two sulfurs that formed the disulfide bridge. This leaves only one sulfur to hold each hair together. Now composed of only half of the sulfurs it previously had, this bond is structurally weak. Before the chemicals were applied, there were two partners holding each hair together. Now there's just one lonely bond left to keep it together.

The remaining sulfur forms a new type of bond, called a lanthionine bond. Once lanthionine bonds have formed, they are irrevocable; the chemical content of your hair has been irreversibly changed, so it's no

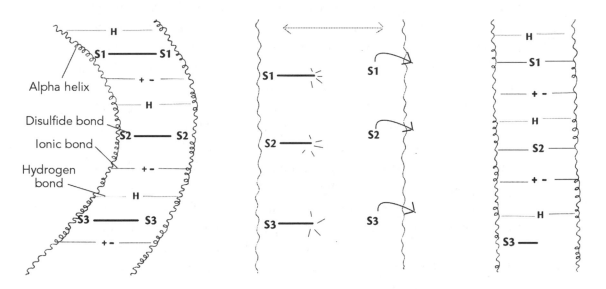

How hydroxides relax your hair.

Before relaxing:

All bonds are present.

During relaxing:

In the highly alkaline environment all H and ionic bonds are broken. Most disulfide bonds are broken and one sulfur from each bond is lost. Hair swells greatly and softens. It can now be molded into a new shape.

After relaxing:

The remaining sulfur now forms a weaker lanthionine link in place of the stronger disulfide bond. Not all bonds form again.

longer the same hair you started with. After the bonds are widowed, they can't bond with other partners. Because these new bonds are much weaker than before, as a result, your altered hair is now weak, with little elasticity remaining.

In addition to undermining the inherent strength of your hair, these caustic chemicals can easily burn your skin and (as I found out) can dissolve your hair. Leaving these chemicals on for only one minute longer than the recommended time can cause increasingly severe damage to your hair. The chemicals will weaken it to the point that your hair breaks easily, even from everyday combing.

Once your cuticles are sticking up from this damage, it's easy to tear them away during normal brushing and styling. This hair is now overly porous, and with no protection, it splits and breaks easily. With your cuticles open, more water can get into the cortex, so it swells when you wash your hair but becomes drier and drier each time because it can no longer hold the moisture in. Once the cortex is exposed, it quickly unravels and practically explodes. At worst, these chemicals can dissolve or partially dissolve your hair. Then nothing can bring it back. The only thing you can do is cut off what's left and start over again.

If your hair is repeatedly processed, the areas on your hair where different procedures took place can overlap. Your hair fibers in those overlapping areas might be so weak they simply shatter and fall apart. Every time your hair is permed or relaxed, bonds are lost. At some point and after repeated perms, there might be few bonds left to hold your hair together anymore. Your hair then breaks into millions of little pieces. Due to my use of relaxers, this was what happened to my hair for my entire adolescence. My shirts were constantly covered in little broken hair pieces where my strands simply were too weak to hold together, and my hair fell apart by the thousands.

Never the Two Shall Meet

Because the chemicals used in straighteners (and perms or curly perms as well) and relaxers change your hair in different ways, the two chemicals should *never* come in contact with each other on the same head of hair. Never use relaxers on straightened or permed hair, and never use straighteners or perms on relaxed hair. Using both on the same hair could potentially break down all of the bonds that were set up by one or the other. Chemically, the second process wouldn't be able to put the bonds back together again that the first process broke. Your hair would then literally disintegrate. If you're set on using chemicals on your hair, it's crucial to strand-test your hair before applying any chemicals to it. It's far less devastating to dissolve a test strand of hair than to use your entire head of hair as a test patch and dissolve it.

Curlocide

I used to think hair products worked by some sort of magic. I believed that the contents in my perms and coloring bottles always knew what to do. I believed that I simply needed to find the right one, and my hair would be transformed. While searching for the right product to work its wonders, I went through many heads of hair.

Now that I understand what the chemicals actually do and how they do it, as well as what they can't do, I have much more respect for the power within those bottles. I now know there never was a magic bullet in any product. It turns out that understanding my hair and treating it humanely was the magic bullet I'd been searching for all along.

I finally realized, after all these years, why my hair constantly broke off in pieces. Not only was I using hydroxide chemicals on my hair, but I was also applying them incorrectly. My hair was breaking off because the bonds holding it together had been destroyed. Maybe if my individual hairs were thicker, they might have survived the chemicals. But they weren't. Areas were probably partially eaten away from the depilatory-like chemicals, so there was little left to hold the hairs together. Strands of my hair fell apart like tissue paper in the rain. I now know that from the moment I smeared that burning cream onto my hair, my hair was doomed.

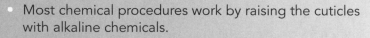

- Most chemical procedures work by raising the cuticles with alkaline chemicals.

- Drastically lightening your hair causes severe damage.

- There are two basic types of perms: those that use thioglycolate and others that employ some form of hydroxide.

- Hair straighteners use thioglycolate. It's relatively mild, although it still damages your hair.

- Hair relaxers use hydroxides, the same types of chemicals that are found in hair removers and drain cleaners.

- Relaxing drastically changes the chemical composition of your hair. This process is highly damaging.

- Never overlap a relaxer with a straightener. You could lose your hair.

Chapter Thirteen

How to Do Your 'Do
The Style Gallery

Our hair looks like no one else's hair. Just as our hair can look unhappy and stiff when we relax it, when straight hair is permed to look curly, it doesn't have the same presence as a crown of jubilant natural spirals and twists. Our hair isn't more difficult to style than other hair types are; it simply needs to be treated differently. Whereas people with straight hair must spend time brushing their hair into place, anchoring it firmly so that it doesn't come undone, and sometimes coating the whole thing in sprays and gels so that it stays put, we can simply swirl our curls into a shape, use one or two pins to anchor it into place, and we're done. Styling our curls in a way that enhances and plays up our texture will make the most of our hair's uniqueness.

Sometimes it's difficult to think of new hairstyles every day, and it's easy to get in a rut. Most of the time, instructions for how to create a particular style are meant for straighter hair. Almost all of the instructions I see (including those that say they're for tightly curled hair) include brushing it. If we brushed our tight curls, we'd be trying to style a fuzzball instead of curls. I love the look of my hair when it's big (so long as the curls are separated by finger combing to prevent damage rather than dry brushing or dry combing). It's just that there are times when I may prefer curls, and it's nice to have options. I know I sound like a broken record, but you should never brush or comb your dry curls. If you do, you won't have curls anymore, and you will most likely damage your hair in the process.

It's a misconception that little can be done with curly hair. In fact, curls are easy to style. They need minimal fastening to keep them in place, and I've never used hairspray in my life. Our curls add interest and texture to any style simply by the grace of their presence. If height is needed, we only have to arrange our hair higher, and height is automatically there. At most, we need only to finger-comb our hair to give it extra thickness in a spot, unlike straighter hair, which needs very damaging backcombing or teasing. And as you know, our hair is built for drama! It's time we took advantage of its dramatic nature. We need to view this as an asset, rather than a liability. The "Exotics" section of this chapter has ideas for playing up the striking feats that only very curly hair can accomplish.

The styles in this book are to be used only as rough guidelines. I did all of them totally by myself and spent a couple of minutes on each one. I didn't use any styling products in these pictures, either. At the most, I used a little conditioner to smooth down any extra fuzz. I didn't have the help of stylists to make sure each style was perfect, so you know the styles shown here don't need a team to create them. I'm not a stylist (and am, in fact, rather uncoordinated), so the fact that I can manage these styles is proof that they are easy. Without help, I am not smooth enough to pull off a complicated style. I am also somewhat lazy and easily distracted, so if a style takes too long, I'm not going to bother. Or else I will wander off and start to do something else.

Ways to Mix Up the Styles

You can use all of these suggested styles as basic templates and add to each one however you like. Some ideas for the styles to give them variety are to use ribbons, pretty clips, and barrettes and pins, as well as hair sticks and hair covers. You can clip up the front of your hair to add height.

Ribbons

Instead of merely pulling your hair back with a coated rubber band for your ponytail, you could tie a pretty ribbon over the rubber band and finish it in a bow. The ribbon would instantly take your ponytail from standard to romantic and lovely.

Pretty Clips, Barrettes, Pins, and Hair Sticks

Decorative clips or barrettes can enhance any of these styles. You could use one to pull the hair off your face in front. Many barrettes are available enameled or in glass, with beads or sparkly rhinestones in lovely colors. You can also get interesting shapes, such as flowers or dragonflies, ranging in size from tiny to large. Subtle ones would add more interest to your hair without calling attention to them. You could also look for bobby pins with a flower, a gemstone, or a sparkly decoration on the end to pin back your hair or even distribute them throughout your curls, especially if your hair is swept up into a romantic bun or pinned up off your neck. I can think of few things lovelier than a beautiful flower nestled into a glossy cascade of curls.

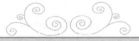

Your Curly Gift

When I was a student at UCSC, there was a young woman with hair much like Aja's (see chapter 6), who wore a lovely fresh flower behind her ear every day. I loved to see her. It was like her beauty was a gift. View your stunning curls as a gift you give to the world by honoring them and treating them like the works of art that they are.

Hair sticks are fun to decorate any of the bun styles. There are some lovely ones out there, from those intricately carved from wood or bone to beaded sticks, to sterling silver with bezel-set gems, to simple smooth faux-tortoiseshell sticks.

You can also use a gorgeous brooch in your hair. Your thick curly hair is the only kind of hair that can support the weight of a precious-metal brooch pinned in it. Take advantage of it!

Clipping Up the Front to Add Height to Your Style

Almost all of the styles I suggest are the simplest versions possible. This means you can add lots of individual touches to them. Try taking some of your front hair and clipping it back, near the front of your crown. This adds drama to your style. Because your hair is thick, it can be scrunched up high and clipped that way. You can easily turn your curls into art by using a pretty barrette or lovely clips to add height and give even more detail to your curls, which are already rich with texture. (I call this "the Elaine" because it looks like how the character Elaine—played by Julia Louis-Dreyfus on the television show *Seinfeld*—used to pin up her hair.)

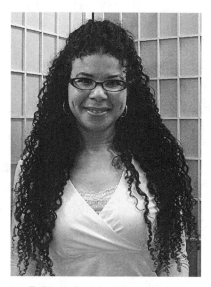

I call this style "the Elaine."

Wear Your Hair Loose

There are many ways to vary this basic style. You could clip one or both sides of your hair back with lovely clips. You could make a side part and then sweep half of your hair off your face and clip it back. You can use a pretty ribbon or a headband to keep your hair pulled back during the day.

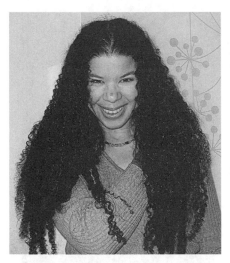

The basic loose style.

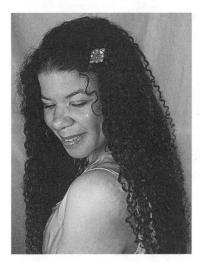

My hair down, with a brooch functioning as a barrette.

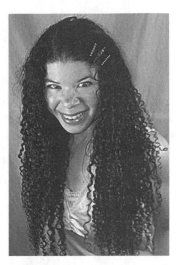

Two barrettes and one brooch holding my hair back.

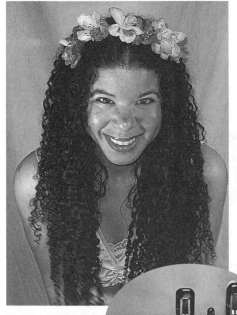

Rhododendrons in my hair.

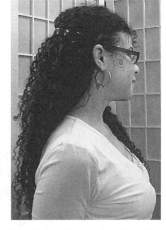

The front clipped back with a hair clip.

I fastened in each flower with a simple snap barrette.

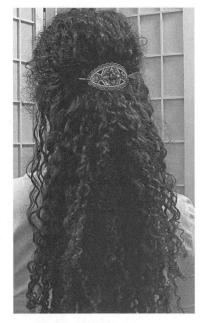

The front pinned back with a barrette.

Ways to Wear Your Hair Partly Loose

- The front clipped up and the rest down (see photos page 223 and at right)
- The front in a half-tail and the rest down (see "Half-Tails")
- The front tied in a knot in the back, with half down (see "Knots")
- The front tied in a knot on top of your head, with half down (see "Knots")
- Half up in a French twist and half down (see "French Twist")
- Half up in a simple twist and half down (see "Simple Twist")
- The front in a bun, with half down (see "Buns")

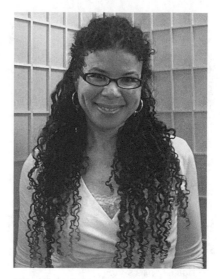

For this style, I used a clip that you can pinch open. I gathered the front of my hair to the back, slid the clip in place, and released it.

Easy Wet-Setting

When I was a teenager, I spent many miserable hours trying to learn to put my thick wet hair in rollers in hopes of making it look straight. It never worked. I'm just not that coordinated. Plus, I don't have the time or patience to neatly put in all of those rollers. Besides that, I can't sleep in those things anyway, and I always feel kind of ridiculous wearing them. But that's beside the point. Thousands of salons, books, magazines, and products out there are clamoring to straighten our curls, one way or another. The purpose of this book is to show you how to care for the curls you were born with. That's why this book is filled with styles for our curls, not for broken-spirited, straightened hair.

Yet this is one technique I use that won't damage your hair to get it straighter. It will not be bone straight. None of the styles here are for straight hair. As I said, you have the rest of the world to help you with that. Having straight hair requires skills I don't have and am not interested in learning. Our curls are unique, and they're spectacular when we show them off. There's so much straight hair already out there; I don't want to contribute to that trend. I do understand, however, that there might be occasions when you'd like to have wavier, rather than curlier, hair. Although I felt like I was cheating on my hair (due to the past we've had together) doing this style for the book, here's my technique for making your curls wavier.

Setting Waves with Two-Stranded Twists

As I mentioned in chapter 10, this is the set to use when you're growing out a relaxer. When you set both types of hair (straight and very curly) in twists, it hides their difference. It's sort of a meeting ground between two opposing textures.

Two-stranded twists make spirals. The smaller your sections, the tighter the wave or spiral pattern, and the firmer the set will stay in your hair. You'll need the following:

- Clips to hold your hair out of your way
- Optional: Clips to hold the ends of your hair together if the ends have been straightened
- A spray bottle filled with water
- A little conditioner to put on your ends to keep the ends curled together
- A little setting lotion or moisturizing gel (they're usually needed only to keep straightened ends together)

To make your twists, first take about a one-inch section of your hair and pin back the rest. Finger-comb the section out gently; start by unraveling the ends and carefully working upward. When that section is big and puffy, mist it with water. You can use a little setting lotion or gel if you feel ambitious. Beware of having your hair too wet when you set it. Air can't get in to dry it out, so make sure it is only barely damp. Then divide the one-inch section in half and twist the two halves around each other to the ends. When you're done, unpin your hair, get another section to work on, and do the same to it. When one section is done, move to the next one. An average number of twists is about twenty. Feel free to make more or fewer of them to vary the tightness of your set. If you're growing out a relaxer, the ends of your hair might be too straight to stay together the way natural curls do. You can clip the ends to keep them in place while they dry, if necessary. Then for sleeping, remove the clips and pull your twists up into a few buns. (Either that, or set your almost-dry hair in about six braids—three braids on each side of your head—to keep your ends together.)

Sleep on your twists overnight. Make sure your hair is dry before undoing them. When you undo them in the morning, always be careful of the ends—they will tangle. Hold the very tips of your hair as you undo the twist or the braid. When you reach the ends, either loosen your hold slightly on the ends so that they can finish spiraling open between your fingers, or untwist only your ends, holding onto them firmly. (You can see how I do this in chapter 10.) Once the sections are undone, finger-comb lightly to fluff them up, or finger-comb them heavily for a more impressive, full look.

To keep this style, put your hair in a bun or a braid at night. *Don't mist in the morning.* When you undo your braid or bun, your waves should still be there. Because you set them damp, they become your hair's default set until they get wet again. As the week goes on, you'll find that your hair gets bigger and less "set" looking. I like the big look, but if it bothers you, you can mist and reset your hair every night in twists. This is more time-consuming, but it will keep your set firm.

Setting Waves with French Braids

Braids make flat waves, while the two-stranded twists make spirals. To make braids, first take half of your hair and pin back the rest. Finger-comb the first half out gently; start by unraveling the ends and carefully working upward. When that section is big and puffy, mist it with water. You can use a little setting lotion or gel if you feel ambitious. Then French braid that half of your hair. Unpin the other half, and do the same to it. Sleep on it overnight. Beware of having your hair too wet when you put it in a braid, because air can't get in to dry it out. Because of this, make sure your hair is only slightly damp when it's put into a braid.

You could also create this look by making two to four regular braids on each half of your head. Regular braids might be easier to do than French braids, which I struggled with (lots of tangling opportunities with all those divisions for the French braids). The important thing is to make sure that all of your hair is included in the braid so it can become set.

Sleep on your braids. In the morning when you undo them, always be careful of the ends. The ends will tangle. Hold the very tips of your hair as you undo your braids. When you reach the end, either loosen your hold slightly on the ends so they can finish spiraling open between your fingers, or untwist only your ends, holding onto them firmly. Once the sections are undone, finger-comb lightly to fluff them up, or finger-comb them heavily for a more impressive, full look.

To keep this style, finger-comb out any snarls at night, re-spritz with water or use setting lotion, and braid again. Another option is to put your hair in a bun or two at night. This will further loosen the waves, so, as the week goes on, your hair will look straighter and fuller. I find that this style gets fuzzy faster than curls do, because your hair doesn't have the security of other

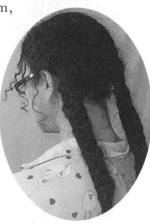

This is how I set my hair for the wavy hair photos below.

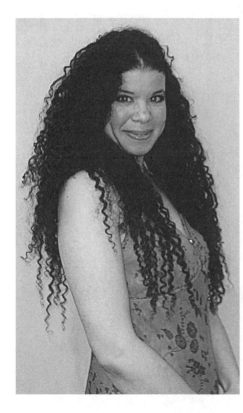

My hair set in waves. To tell you the truth, I think the waves look a bit like I'm wearing a weave. And, to be honest, after all those years of hurting my curls, I felt guilty wearing my hair in waves, rather than in my natural curls.

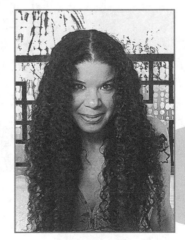

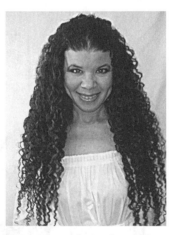

Set waves with the front of my hair pinned back.

If you wanted a smoother look, at night you could put your hair back in a bun or a braid, which would flatten the waves out even more than this.

curls to curl with. And like straightened hair, set styles puff up with humidity. Yet this also causes the style to be even more impressive-looking. Few people have big, thick manes of hair, so enjoy yours in all the ways you are able to wear it.

Easy-to-Do Ponytail Styles

Ponytail styles are about the easiest to do, and they work for medium-length hair or longer. Here are a few of the styles I wear my hair in. They are great for when I'm running late in the morning because they take only seconds to do.

The Basic Ponytail

A simple ponytail is an all-purpose standby. It's a great style when you don't have time to think of anything else. There are so many variations for this look, depending on where you place the tail. Placing your ponytail low

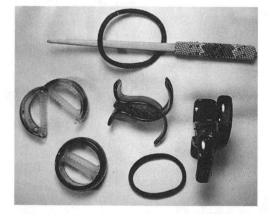

Various types of hair holders. Always use bands that are covered with fabric, and double-check that there are few snagging parts to catch in your hair.

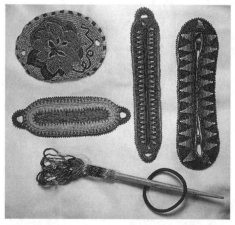

Handmade beaded barrettes. When I was first growing out my hair, it got so big I had to make barrettes to fit it.

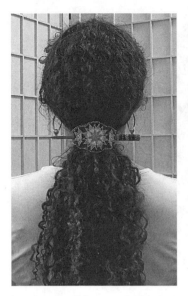

Low ponytail fastened with a beaded barrette.

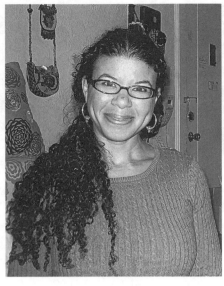

Low ponytail from the front.

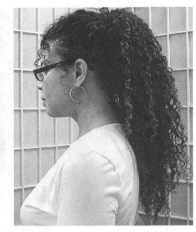

High ponytail fastened with a clip.

and loose is a very romantic look. A low but firm ponytail has a sort of ballerina look to it. It would be beautiful with a ribbon tied into a crisp bow over the band. Ponytails look sporty positioned near the middle or high on your head. If you have shorter hair and wear your ponytail nearly at the top of your head so that your curls spill down on either side, it gives you a lovely, happy crown of spirals framing your face.

Remember to never pull your hair so tight that it's stretching your face to the sides. This will not only torture and break your hair, but it could cause massive hair loss at your hairline.

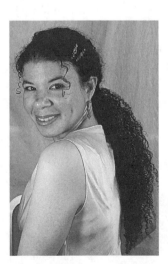

Ponytail with two brooches as barrettes.

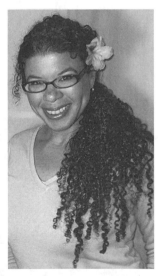

Ponytail with a flower.

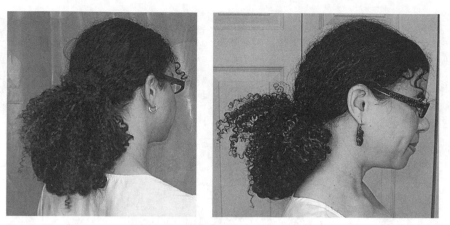

The half-tail from the back and the side.

Half-Tail

This is another good standby style; it's great for work if your job tends to be active or hectic. This style keeps your ends out of the way.

How to make a half-tail.

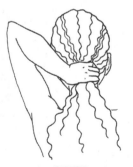

Gather all your hair back into a ponytail in your hand.

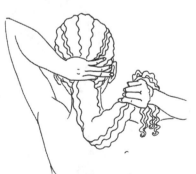

Take the ends and bring them up to the base of your ponytail.

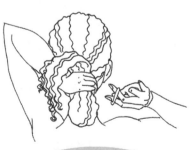

Put a band around folded hair, or clip it.

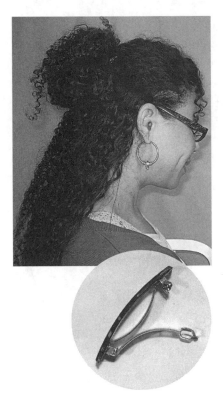

Half-Tail and Loose

This is a variation of the half-tail. It's a great way to keep your hair out of your face in a fun style, without having to put much work into it. To make it, divide your hair in half from ear to ear. Take the top half and put it into a half-tail (see figure on page 130). Then you're done!

I fastened the half-tail with a barrette. I took the middle section out so that the clip would fit my hair (see below).

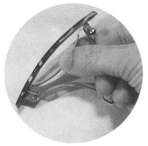

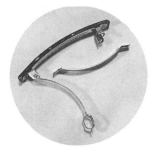

You can give your hair more breathing room in your standard barrette by removing the center bar. It comes out easily, and you can always put it back in if you need to.

The center bar has been taken out. There is now a bit more room in the barrette for your hair to fit.

Girdle Tail

This is a variation on the half-tail. It is useful if your hair is long enough that it still hangs low, even with the half-tail. I can't do half-tails easily anymore because part of it still hangs low enough that it catches behind my back when I sit. Then when I try to look down—for instance, to type at my computer—I can't because my hair has gotten trapped between my back and the chair.

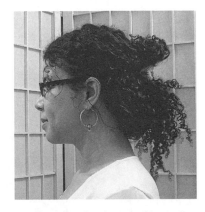

Girdle tail with a beaded barrette.

This is a great style to show off a lovely barrette. Styling your hair in a half-tail when you have long hair means that the ends of your hair will cover the barrette you use. So if you have a barrette you'd like to show off, the girdle tail is the style to try. The girdle tail also has an Asian or almost Native American look to it. It would be great with a beaded barrette and turquoise earrings.

How to make a girdle tail.

Gather your hair in a ponytail. Twist it lightly once or twice for a looser tail. Twist it all the way to the ends for a firmer tail.

While keeping the twist anchored at the base with one hand, bring up the ends of your hair to the top of your head.

Fold over your ends and clip them down, so your curls face downward.

Customized hair band: If your hair is so thick you can't use a basic store-bought barrette, here's a trick to pull up your hair. You can use a fabric-covered band (such as those found in the hair-care sections of drugstores or beauty supply stores) or even a stretchy headband and a hair stick to create a customized band. Put your hair in the desired style, such as the girdle tail or the half-tail. Then take the band and stretch it over the area you would normally have fastened with the barrette. Use a hair stick (or even a pencil or a chopstick), and insert it into your band, under your hair, and out the other side of the band (see the picture at right).

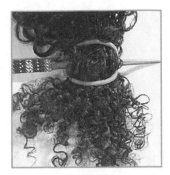

Customized hair band using a regular fabric-covered hair band and a hair stick.

Braids

Braids are a great all-purpose style. They're perfect for sleeping, swimming, traveling, and downpours. When your hair is drying, and you have to perform an activity that could mess it up, nothing battens down your hair hatches like a nice firm braid or two.

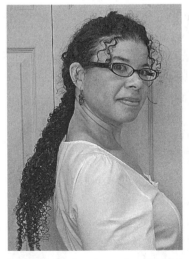

A braid with loose ends, with the front of the hair clipped back.

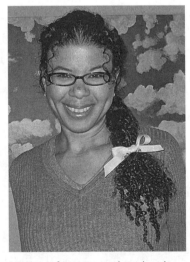

You can fasten your braid with a ribbon for a lovely look.

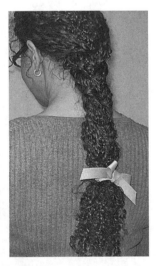

A braid and a bow from the back.

How to make a basic braid

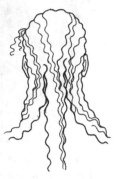

Divide your hair into three sections.

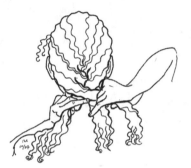

Braid your hair by crossing the outer section over the section closest to it, alternating sides.

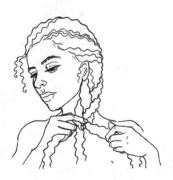

Braid loosely, and stop about three-quarters of the way down. For curly hair, you probably don't need to fasten the ends.

You can make a firm braid for functional use, or you can make a very loose, romantic braid. Depending on your curl, you might not need to secure the ends. Or you could secure them with a lovely bow tied near the ends to hold them.

Two Braids (Good for Travel)

Two braids are great for traveling. The bulk of your hair will be on either side of your head, so any rubbing or wear and tear on your hair is minimized. Rubbing usually happens directly in the back of your head when it's leaning against the seat. This is also another heavy-duty style for swimming. It keeps your hair firmly in place so that there's minimal tangling, plus it's already divided in half so you can take each braid down one at a time to comb it.

Back in my teenage years, when I wore my hair texturized, my family went on a twelve-hour trip. I was so afraid of my hair matting that I didn't once let my head touch the back of the seat. So I couldn't sleep unless I rested my face on my hand, which I wouldn't do because I knew that touching my face would make it break out worse. Needless to say, I was pretty crabby by the time we arrived.

Flower-Child Braids (or Twists)

This style always looks so lovely and carefree, almost as if you can see flowers braided into your strands of hair. Our hair is perfect for this style because it holds its shape so well. You can put just your front hair into braids or twists and then tie or clip them back for a gorgeous bohemian look.

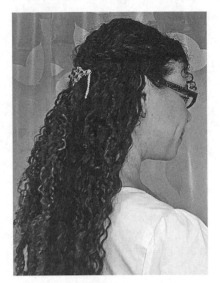

The front of my hair in two twists, fastened with a barrette.

You can also create this look by pinning or braiding or wearing the remainder of your hair in a ponytail. This gives your hair even more visual interest.

Styles to Make with Braids

- Two braids
- A braid bun
- Two braids in front, tied or clipped back, with hair down
- Two braids in front, tied or clipped back, with a braid
- Two braids in front, tied or clipped back, with a ponytail
- Two braids in front, tied or clipped back, with a bun

Knots

Knots are a great way to show off your quirky hair. Because it loves to grab and hold onto things, why not take advantage of its nature? If you're wearing your hair loose and you get tired of it falling into your face, you can take the front hair and tie it back into a knot—and it stays. You can also tie your hair in a knot at the top of your head to add lots of drama and height to your style within minutes.

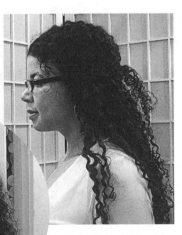

The sides tied in a knot.

Side view of the sides tied in a knot.

How to tie your hair back with a knot.

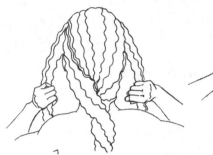 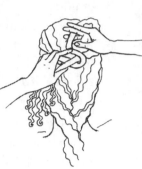 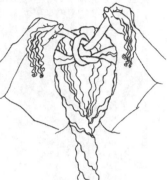

Separate two pieces from the front of your hair.

Wrap one end under the other.

Now take the other end and tie it over the first, making a knot. Tighten it gently.

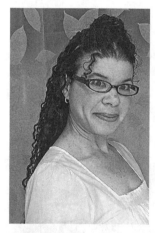

A knot tied at the top of my head, with the rest of my hair loose. I fastened the knot with the same kind of pin that I use for buns.

Styles You Can Make with Knots

- A knot on top of your head, with the rest of your hair loose or in a ponytail, a braid, or a bun.
- Tied back with a low ponytail.
- Tied back with a braid.
- Tied back with a bun.
- Two braids tied back into a knot; the rest of your hair loose, in a bun, a braid, or a ponytail.

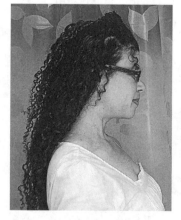 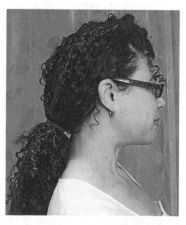

Side view of the front of my hair in a knot.

A knot on top of my head, the rest of my hair in a ponytail.

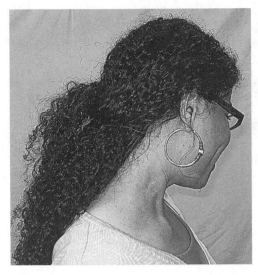

Most of my hair tied in a single knot. First, I divided my hair into three sections. Then I took the sections on either side of my head and tied them once, leaving the middle section loose.

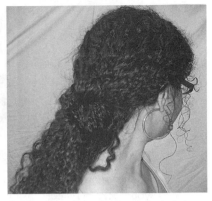

Back view of the bulk of my hair in a knot. This is the same knot; I simply tied it one more time to make it a double knot.

- Two twists tied back into a knot; the rest of your hair loose, in a bun, a braid, or a ponytail.
- You can also tie most of your hair in a single or double knot (see the photos above). Divide your hair into thirds. Take the two sections above your ears and tie them together once or twice.

Buns

This was a style I couldn't pull off back when I was using a relaxer. When I tried to swirl my hair back into a bun, most of the broken strands of my hair stuck straight out, and I couldn't find enough bobby pins to keep them all pinned into the bun. Now I just swirl my hair around a few times and anchor it, often without even looking.

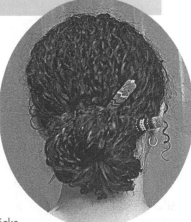

A basic bun with beaded hair sticks.

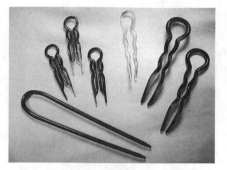

Use from one to four pins to hold your locks in place. Pins function more as anchors than to hold back lots of loose hairs.

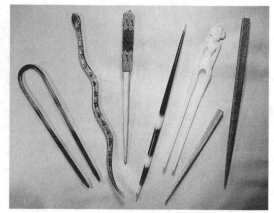

You can decorate your bun with hair sticks.

Basic Bun

Buns are a good, all-purpose style that's perfect for days when you need to protect your hair. They're great for when you're cleaning or painting, for very rainy days, when you haven't had a chance to comb your hair, or when you simply want to put it up out of the way. They are also an understated and elegant style for work. You can also put your hair in one or two buns for sleeping. Use simple tortoiseshell pins or a long U-shaped pin and decorate the bun with chopsticks.

How to make a basic bun.

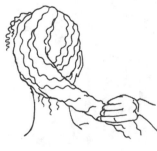

Gather your hair back and twist.

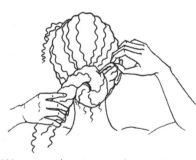

Wrap your hair in a circle, pinning it near the top of the turn.

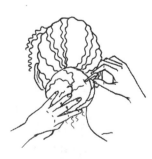

Tuck in the ends and pin again.

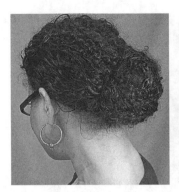

A braid bun with the front clipped up.

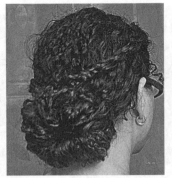

A bun with the front hair in two twists that are then put into the bun.

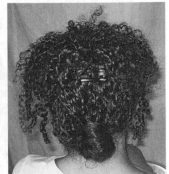

A bun with the ends left loose and clipped near the top of the head.

Basic Bun Variations

These are done much like a regular bun. For the braid bun, you braid your hair first, then swirl it up into a bun and pin it. For the bun with two twists, you twist the front of your hair first, then pull your hair into a regular bun. For the bun-up, swirl your hair once around as if you were making a bun, then clip the ends instead of tucking them.

Romantic Bun

This bun looks complicated, but with our particular hair, it's easy to do. It's perfect for a wedding if you drape it with strings of pearls or tiny clear crystals or tuck flowers into it.

Several versions of romantic buns.

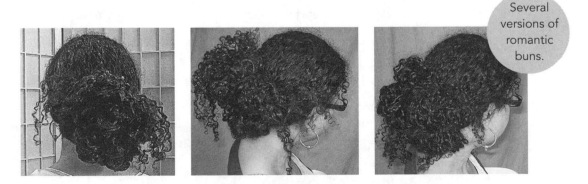

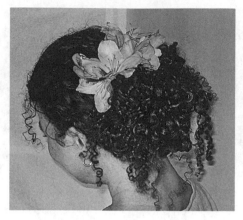
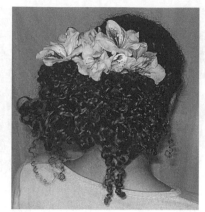

The romantic bun with flowers pinned on top.

The romantic bun with flowers, shown from the back.

How to make a romantic bun.

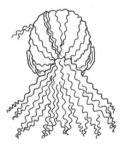
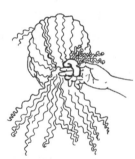
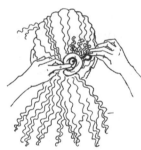
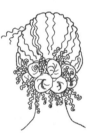

Pull your hair back into a loose ponytail.

Take a section of your hair and make a loose loop around your fingers. For longer hair, wrap the loop around your fingers twice.

Pin curl into place, leaving ends out.

Repeat this about seven or more times, until all your hair has been loosely pinned up.

Figure-8 Bun

This bun also looks complicated, but once you understand how to do it, you can make it in less than two minutes. Its beauty is that it looks sophisticated, as if it took a long time to create. In reality, it can be whipped together in no time.

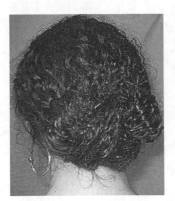

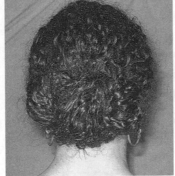

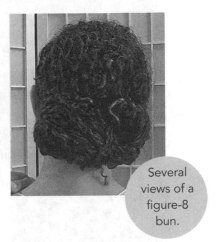

Several views of a figure-8 bun.

How to make a figure-8 bun.

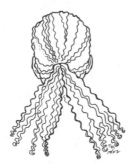

1. Start with your hair in a ponytail. Divide ponytail in half.

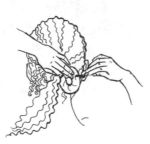

2. Take one half of your ponytail and begin to loop it in a figure 8. Pin as you go.

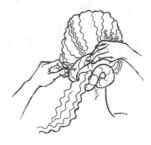

3. Loop figure 8 under the loose half of your hair.

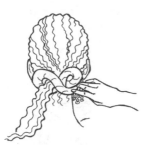

4. Finish the figure 8 by tucking it in and pinning.

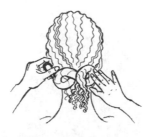

5. Make another figure 8 with the other half. Wrap it over the first figure 8. Pin as you go.

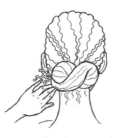

6. Tuck in the ends and pin.

Double Bun

This is a fun style that's not only easy to do, but very secure. The hardest part is deciding where to divide the two halves of hair. A hair stick through both buns helps to unify them but isn't necessary. This is the perfect style for you to wear all kinds of lovely and quirky hair sticks with.

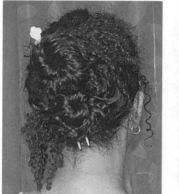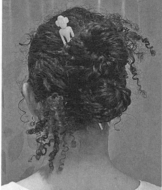

A double bun with a monkey-man hair stick.

Bun and Loose

Any of these buns would look great combined with loose hair. Divide your hair in half from ear to ear. Choose one of the bun styles for the top half of your hair. Leave a few tendrils loose or the entire bottom half of your hair down.

The front of my hair in a basic bun with hair sticks, the rest down.

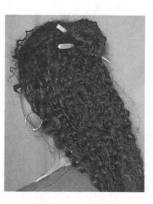

How to make a double bun.

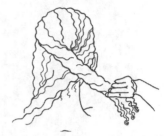

Divide your hair roughly in half, from ear to ear. Take the top half and twist it.

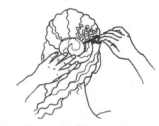

Wrap the top half into a bun. Leave the ends loose and pin.

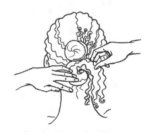

Twist the bottom half into a bun and pin, again leaving the ends loose.

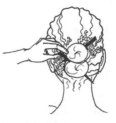

For added interest, decorate with chopsticks.

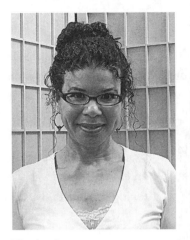

The basic ant.

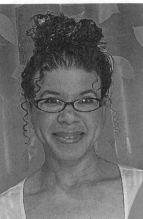

An ant at the top of my head.

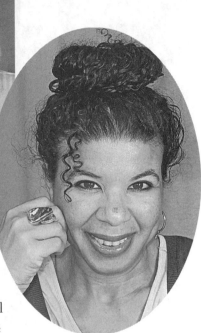

The ant is versatile. It can make you look businesslike and efficient if you're going to a corporate job interview—or you can use one to get your hair out of the way before taking a bath.

African Ant

My mom named this style based on old cartoons featuring African ant characters that wore their hair in a style that looked like this. This style is a basic bun, moved to the top of your head. It's a casual look that keeps your hair out of mischief when you're taking a bath or going to a sauna. To give it volume, put your head upside down, gather all of your hair at the top of your head (the bigger your hair, the better), and swirl it loosely into a big bun. I usually secure it with only one long U-shaped pin to make it even more casual.

Easy-to-Do Twist Styles

Twist styles range from fun to elegant. The French twist and the French roll take some coordination, but in return they are sturdy and sophisticated.

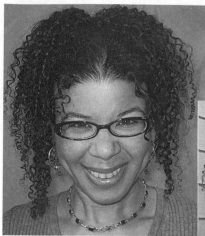

Simple Twist

This is basically a French twist with the ends left loose instead of tucked in. It has the elegance of a French twist, but your curls spill out on top. It's easier to do than a French twist because you don't have to worry about tucking in your ends.

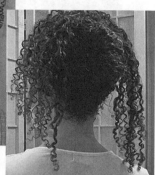

The twist was fastened using a large hair clip.

The same twist, but from the back.

In these photos, especially the side view photo, you can see all of the different sizes of curls I have. I know that the techniques in this book work for every kind of curl because I grow all types of curls.

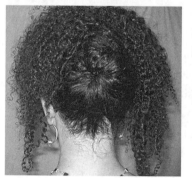

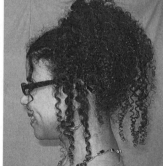

How to make a simple twist.

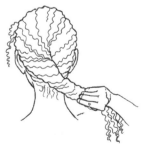

Gather your hair back and twist it.

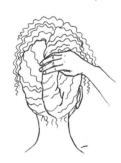

Bring up the twist until the ends are on top of your head.

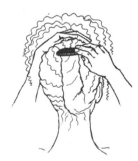

Clip your hair up with a large barrette, a clip, or a hair holder with stick.

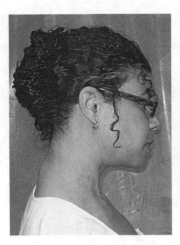

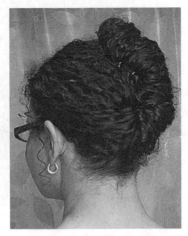

A French twist from the side.

A French twist from the back.

French Twist

Nothing beats the sophistication of a French twist. This is a style that I always wanted to wear as a child. I'd hear about someone wearing a "French twist," and it always sounded so mysterious and elegant. Yet no one around me at the time knew how to make one. In my teenage years, the few instructions I read were vague, and I still wasn't sure how to make French twists. Once I figured out how they were done, they were easy. You do need to keep your eyes on the top of your head because the hair there can get lumpy, so you have to take extra care to tuck it in and pin it.

French Roll Method

This is a variation of the French twist. When it's done, it looks much like the basic French twist (see above). The difference is that for the French twist, you twist up your hair and tuck in the ends.

How to make a French twist.

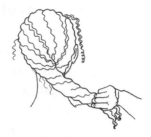

Gather your hair back and twist it.

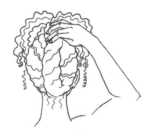

Bring the twist up so that your ends are resting on the top of your head.

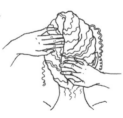

Fold the ends over and tuck them under the twist. Roll the twist slightly toward the ends and tuck it until firm.

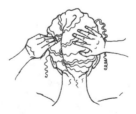

Pin it in place with about four pins.

The French roll starts out easy, but tucking in your ends can be a challenge. The roll takes a bit more coordination to start, but the ends are rolled in from the beginning, so when you're finished rolling it, you're done.

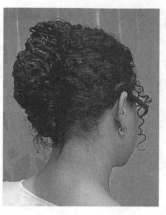

A French roll from the right side.

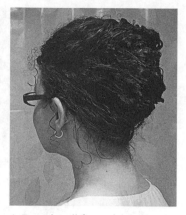

A French roll from the left side.

How to make a French roll.

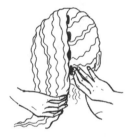

Pin back half your hair using about four clips.

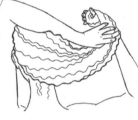

Take the loose half of your hair and roll it to the middle.

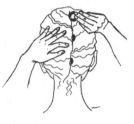

Tuck in any loose ends and puffy parts.

Pin the roll in place using about four pins.

French Twist with Loose Hair

Part your hair in two, from ear to ear. Take the top half and make a French twist with it (either the twist or the roll method is fine, whichever is easiest for you). Leave the rest loose for a sophisticated look.

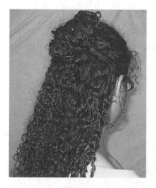

A French roll as it looks from the right side.

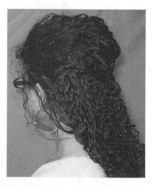

And the same roll from the left side.

Exotics

These are the styles that play up the drama and holding ability of your hair. All those years I felt that my hair embarrassed me by transforming into a big rain cloud around my head can now be turned to my advantage. Nothing makes an entrance like walking into a room with a giant mane of hair wider than your shoulders. Show off that volume! And what about long twists hanging down your back that could never quite be duplicated by extensions and that straighter hair couldn't hold together without clunky rubber bands?

Big Hair

This style takes advantage of your hair's tendency to expand. Depending on the length and tightness of your curl, this look will get lots of attention. There are few things more dramatic than seeing someone enter a room with a huge cloud of hair. This style fills doorways, and it's hard to ignore.

It takes some time to create big hair in a way that avoids damaging your hair, so be careful. For the biggest hair, you need to have dry curls. Take one curl at a time, and gently pull it apart with your fingers. Do this until your entire head is undone. It's best to stop an inch or two from the ends. This prevents your ends from turning into a mat by the end of the evening. If you want, run your fingers over each end to loosen its curl, while still keeping it intact. This gives you huge hair but keeps the ends in their curls to prevent chaos. You can also wet the ends a little to curl them, which gives them a bit of definition.

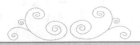

Preparing to Style

If you know ahead of time that you want to do the big-hair style or twists, your best bet is to rinse out most of the conditioner (before or after you comb, depending on how difficult your hair is to comb with most of the conditioner rinsed out), let your hair dry, then separate out your curls. Because the conditioner is used to help your curls clump, you don't need as much of it when your goal is to unclump them to dramatic effect.

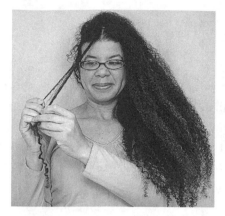

Pulling a curl apart to make big hair. Stop before the end of your curl for more definition on your ends.

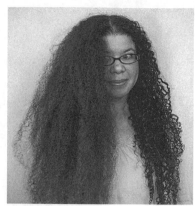

My hair, half big.

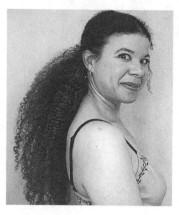

Big hair in a ponytail.

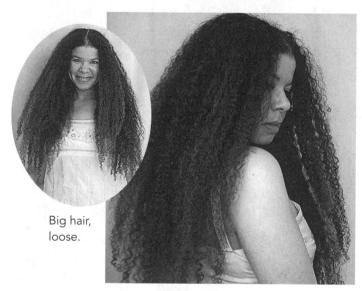

Big hair, loose.

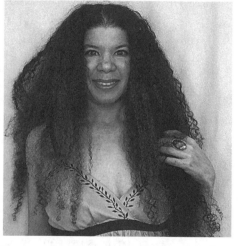

You can see the gossamerlike quality of my hair when the curls have been separated.

Twists

Twists take two or three hours to put in but are worth the effort. Because our hair is so curly, we can put in thicker twists that will stay in our hair without bands to hold the ends together. Because we use our natural hair for this look, we can put in thicker twists that would be difficult to do with extension hair. These twists remind me of photos I've seen of Tibetan women with their long dark twists intricately entwined with colorful beads and coins.

This would also be an excellent style to wear on vacations. Since your hair is divided into bite-size pieces, you could undo a few twists each night to wet, comb through with conditioner, and then re-twist. This holds for swimming as well. If you don't have time during your vacation to sit down and devote two hours in one sitting to combing your hair, twisting it into smaller segments might be perfect. If you're careful, you could even work a bit on your hair anywhere, such as sitting at the beach or in the

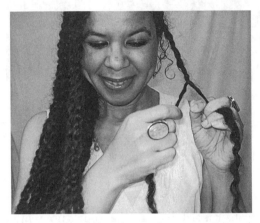

Take two strands and twist them together.

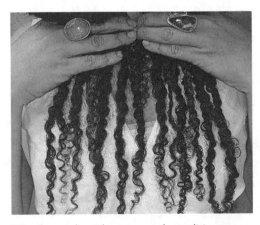

Wet the ends with water and conditioner to define them and keep them in place.

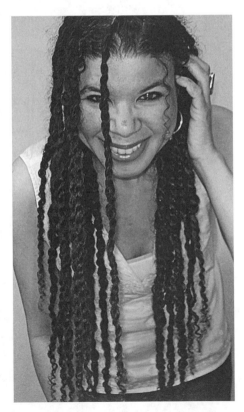

Hair in twists.

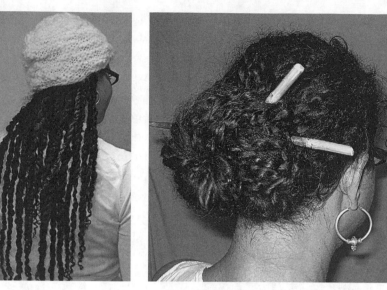

Twists with a hat.   Twists in a bun, with bamboo chopsticks.

airport, by undoing a twist and finger-combing it gently before twisting it back up again.

This style looks best if it's done on dry, finger-combed hair. I've found that if I put the twists in when my hair is still wet, my hair curls up, which makes the twists curl up, break apart into individual curls, and undo themselves.

When you're finished twisting, wet the ends and put a little conditioner on them to make them curl and to protect them. This also helps keep them together, defines them, and lessens tangling.

Special-Occasion Curls

There are certain occasions when you'll want your curls to be photo perfect, and you won't have hours to spend recombing your hair. At times like these, you can refresh your curls to make every spiral flawless. This takes a while, depending on how defined you want your hair to be, but it works wonders.

All that you will need to create amazing curls is water, conditioner, and a few hair clips. Go over your dry hair, curl by curl, and smooth each coil with water and conditioner, just as you do when you set them after combing. Wet your hands, rub some conditioner into your palms, and run your hands down each curl. Replenish the water and conditioner as needed. The more tangled your hair, the more water and conditioner you'll need to smooth it. Try to go in the direction you combed it in. For most of your curls, a run-through with water and conditioner will refresh the spirals and slick down any stray hairs, so that each curl is emphasized. Lift each curl as you smooth it, to make sure it can move freely and hasn't gotten meshed into its neighbors. Lifting the curls as you smooth them will also give them more volume.

Curls near the top of your head, as well as your ends, might need more work. They tend to net together after a few days, so you might need to gently separate each one from the other curls. Once you've freed a tangly curl, run through it with your fingers to reset its hairs, saturating them with water and conditioner to put the curl back together again.

If you find some curls that are really tangled together, you might have to comb a few of them. You may also need to comb any individual curl that doesn't feel smooth when you run your hands down it. Always separate the curl that will be combed from its neighbor curls before you pick up a comb. If you snag other curls with that comb, you'll make lots more work for yourself. And remember, always use water and conditioner every and any time you comb your hair, no matter how small the curl might be.

When you're working at the top of your head, pull up the entire length of each curl as you smooth it. This emphasizes them by causing them to stand away from the rest of your hair a little, showcasing their undulations. Spritz your scalp at your hairline so that your hair plumps and makes your crown even fuller and more lush.

If your hairline is low, you could wet the hair at your forehead, put in a molding paste or a strong gel, and clip it to create deep waves. These will then dry off your face and will add needed height at your temples.

Kapow!

For even more volume, wait until your hair is dry, flip your head upside down, and shake your hair, putting your fingers at the roots and jiggling energetically. Because your hair is eager to express itself in volume, this is often all you need to get impressive body. *Never* backcomb your hair, though. Uncombing backcombed hair is a world of suffering you don't want to visit.

This look can be stunning. You'll have volume and curls for miles. This look is great if you're taking photographs. Since it defines your curls and gives you volume, it will show up well on camera. In fact, this style show-cases what your curls can really do; you can make your hair do things that few other people's hair can. Show off the energy that radiates through your curls. Show them what you've got.

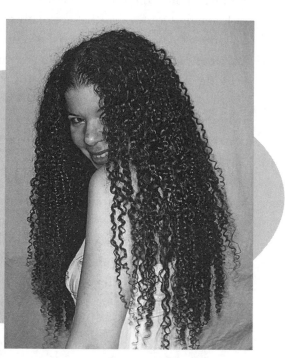

I used the Kapow method for the pictures I took for the cover (this is one of them). To set my hair for the photos, I also wet the front of my hair with water and conditioner, pushed my hair forward, and clipped it up to add height in the front (sort of in an "Elaine"—see earlier in this chapter). I had a big "M" head while the two front mounds of my hair were drying.

- Don't brush your hair to style it. Style it as is.

- Use sturdy, simple fastenings to anchor your hair.

- For any styles that require volume, separate your curls with your fingers, never dry brush or comb your hair.

- For Big Hair, to cut down on tangling, you don't have to separate your curls all the way down to the ends.

- Your hair is unique. Wear it in styles that show off your curls.

Chapter Fourteen

The Philosophy of Curls

I n the process of discovering how to care for my hair, I learned about more than just hair care. When I finally understood what my hair had wanted all along, I was struck by how simple its needs were. It thrives with just a few basic rules of care and rewards me every day with jubilant spirals. By taking what I considered my worst feature and turning it into my best feature, I feel so much better about myself in general. I had wasted so much energy hating my hair and feeling punished by my hair, asking, Why me? Now, this very same hair brings me joy. All that my hair ever wanted was to be itself. How could I deny it a right we should all have?

When I searched for representations of my hair in the media, I found nothing. Even people whose hair looked just like mine were portrayed as having hair that behaves exactly as straight hair does. I began to feel as if my hair fell outside the range of what was "normal." In this isolation, it became easy for me to think my hair was an aberration. My mantra used to be, Why can't it just act like *normal* hair?

When I tried to force my hair to look like everyone else's straighter hair, it was a wretched imitation of their hair. When I let it be itself, it blossomed. Dealing with my hair constructively meant that I had to learn a whole new way to think about it. I needed to approach my hair with understanding and strategy, instead of blindly hacking away at it. Decades of brutality through chemicals and roughness left me with crunchy, broken hair. I lived my life with hair that felt more like an intruder than a part of me. Of course, I had hair that was broken—look what I was doing to it! I tried to see things from my hair's point of view. If hydroxides burned my skin, didn't that mean they were scorching my hair as well? If ripping a brush over my skin made it raw, wouldn't that damage my hair if I did the same to it?

When I decided to accept my hair for the very curly hair that it is, it became a puzzle to solve, rather than a punishment to endure. When I faced the truth for what it was, no matter what, and embraced it, it suddenly wasn't so alien and scary. I'm not saying you'll like the truth you must face, but you'll be able to make the best of it when you do. And often our biggest lessons in life come from the things that cause us the fiercest struggle. Now I don't want straight hair. In fact, sometimes I worry that my hair might straighten out for some reason. I know that if I had straight hair, I would lose a big part of who I am, and I would lose the friends my curls have become.

In M. Scott Peck's *The Road Less Traveled: A New Psychology of Love, Traditional Values and Spiritual Growth*, one of the tenets is that life is hard, but once you make peace with it being a struggle, you transcend the struggle. You no longer spend your energy fruitlessly banging your head against the wall of what things *should* be like. Instead, your energy is freed to work on what to do about the situation and how to make it better.

I used to squeeze my eyes shut at night, in tears, and wish for different hair. I spent hours nearly every time I left the house looking for a product to "cure" my hair. Now I know there are no shortcuts and no magic products. Having long, healthy hair comes from learning to care for it and taking the time to treat it right. Some of my choices require more time and effort, such as not using heat and letting my hair air dry. But because I'm willing to put a little more time into my hair to be certain I'm gentle, it rewards me many times over with long, happy curls. Our struggles often turn into gifts in disguise, depending on how we approach them.

Your curls are like your fingerprints. They are a part of you, and they are exceptional. They're a combination of your own particular genetic legacy and racial heritage. You wear the curls passed down to you from all of the curly ancestors who came before you. Tight curls worn long and proudly are a rarity, because so few people know how to care for them properly. A head full of rich, gleaming spirals is arresting. The owner of such hair owes it to the world to let others enjoy its beauty. I feel a deep joy when I see a person with hundreds of happy corkscrew curls spinning into the air. It's as if they've finally been allowed to be what they've always passionately wanted to be, and they're ecstatic.

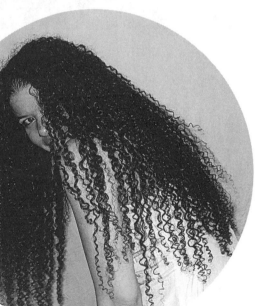

There are so many curly-haired people who have no idea how beautiful healthy curls can be, so they feel that wearing their hair naturally isn't an option. By wearing your spirals, you show others that your hair is beautiful exactly as it grows from your head. You never know; you could inspire someone else to take that leap and embrace his or her own curls, too.

Celebrate your curls' uniqueness.

These are the curls you were born with, and they are a part of you. Curls like yours are a gift that only a special few people have the privilege to grow. Honor them, for they are yours.

Take Away Tips

- Your curls will never act like straighter hair. They will always act like curly hair.

- Throw out notions of how your hair "should" act. Your hair is acting exactly the way curly hair is supposed to.

- There is power in accepting your reality and learning the most constructive way to work *with* it.

- Our struggles often turn into lessons (and gifts) in disguise, depending on how we approach them.

- Why be like everyone else? Celebrate your hair's uniqueness.

- Anything worth having is worth the effort it takes to have. Your beautiful curls are worth the effort.

Recommended Reading

Books

Curly Girl: More Than Just Hair—It's an Attitude: A Celebration of Curls: How to Cut Them, Care for Them, Love Them, and Set Them Free by Lorraine Massey with Deborah Chiel (New York: Workman, 2001). A very curl-friendly book, perfect for people with waves and loose curls. Although this book is primarily for those who have slightly wavy to mildly curly hair (despite what the photos inside indicate), it still has good tips for washing all types of hair that are prone to dryness and frizz, and the book is very curl-positive. It recommends forgoing shampooing altogether and using only conditioner to cleanse. You will need to experiment to see whether this is a good solution for you. I broke out too much when I tried it, but I love the idea. Be aware that it's an option for you.

Don't Go Shopping for Hair Care Products without Me: Over 4,000 Products Reviewed, Plus the Latest Hair-Care Information by Paula Begoun (Seattle: Beginning Press, 2005). I consider this my product bible. It's like having someone demystify the products for you. Begoun tells you the hard truth that will save you money. After reading her book, you'll finally know what you're really buying. It immunizes you against product advertising. The general hair-care information she gives is excellent advice that's true for anyone's hair. Her styling and hair-care tips are geared toward straighter hair than ours, and the African American section has good, standard advice that's true for any hair. Yet although she doesn't give any tips for styling our super-curly hair, her information about ingredients is excellent. In the second half of the book, Begoun decodes the ingredient lists of hundreds of commercially available products. Soon you'll be able to pick up a bottle, flip it over, and know whether it really will condition your hair. After you read this book, it will all become clear. You can also check out her site at www.CosmeticsCop.com.

Going Natural: How to Fall in Love with Nappy Hair by Mireille Liong-A-Kong (New York: Sabi Wiri, 2004). This book is a classic for ideas on how to create intricate, African-inspired styles, such as braids, cornrows, and Afros. Mireille also has a site that's an incredible resource at going-natural.com, as well as a site in Dutch at Kroeshaar.com.

Good Hair: For Colored Girls Who've Considered Weaves When the Chemicals Became Too Ruff by Lonnice Brittenum Bonner (New York: Crown Publishers, 1992). This is the book that inspired me to grow out my relaxer. It's extremely funny and a good read, even if you aren't growing out any chemicals. It's also an excellent book to keep you company while you grow out the chemicals. This book gave me the encouragement I needed to see the difficult growing-out process through. Most of all, the book just cracks me up! Bonner's had about as many hair disasters as I have.

Hair Story: Untangling the Roots of Black Hair in America by Ayana D. Bird and Lori L. Tharps (New York: St. Martin's Press, 2001). I strongly recommend this book to anyone of African descent with curly hair and any parent of a multiracial child of African descent. It's understandably confusing to straighter-haired people why something as simple as hair can be so political to many African Americans. And it's equally difficult to get the answers to why this seems to be such a charged topic. This book explains the history of African American hair in America and gives many of the reasons that hair can be way more than just hair, complete with illustrations.

A Consumer's Dictionary of Cosmetic Ingredients, by Ruth Winter (New York: Three Rivers Press, 2009). This is one of my go-to books when I'm looking up ingredients. Winter is a great resource, especially when I want to find out if an ingredient is considered irritating or is being reexamined for its safety (or lack of it) for inclusion as an ingredient appropriate as a cosmetic.

Black, White, Other: Biracial Americans Talk about Race and Identity by Lise Funderburg (New York: HarperPerennial, 1995). In this book, Funderburg gathers the stories of forty-six mixed-race people who discuss how they view race and how it's affected them. This is a great way to read about the vastly differing experiences of mixed-race people.

Mixed: My Life in Black and White by Angela Nissel (New York: Villard Books, 2006). This is an adult book that vividly describes the conflict the author experienced growing up between two very different worlds. At times it was so funny that I embarrassed myself while reading in public places because I couldn't stop laughing. This book is also bluntly honest, and what she says at times was difficult to read.

Web Sites

This list is by no means exhaustive, but it has a good selection of hair information sites and multiracial sites of all flavors. Most of them have great information, related links, reading lists, communities, and resources:

The Association of MultiEthnic Americans (AMEA) at www.ameasite .org. This site has an extensive reading list of all kinds of books about the multiracial experience.

The Beauty Brains at www.thebeautybrains.com is a wonderful site that helps you cut through all the confusing misinformation out there surrounding our hair products and cosmetics. Written by a group of anonymous cosmetic scientists (anonymous so they can tell you the truth about the different brands without losing their jobs), they tell you the real truth about what's in those products.

Black Girl with Long Hair at http://bglhonline.com/ is a wonderful site filled with so many mouth-watering pictures of beautiful women showing their gorgeous natural curls. The site also discusses natural hair styles, hair products, and hair-care issues.

Curly Nikki at www.curlynikki.com/ is an enthusiastic blog that supports naturally curly hair care and the curly community. Curly Nikki herself has lovely curls, and the site is chock-full of photos of beautiful natural hair.

Interracial Voice at www.webcom.com~intvoice. This site is devoted to multiracial people having their own multiracial identity. It considers itself the "philosophical 'voice of conscience' of the global multiracial community."

Light-skinned-ed girl at http://lightskinnededgirl.typepad.com/my_weblog/. A blog by Heidi Durrow, who always has thought-provoking insights and interesting pictures about her biracial-bicultural experience. She also cohosts "MixedChicksChat," a podcast featuring various mixed-race people and issues.

MAVIN at www.mavin.net. MAVIN is a leading organization that builds healthy communities that celebrate and empower mixed-heritage people and families. Their projects explore the experiences of mixed-heritage people, transracial adoptees, interracial relationships, and multiracial families.

The Mixed Heritage Center at www.MixedHeritageCenter.org. On its site, the center states that it is "a clearinghouse of information relevant to the lives of people who are multiracial, multiethnic, transracially adopted, or otherwise affected by the intersection of race and culture."

The Multiracial Activist at www.multiracial.com. As it says on the home page, this group is "dedicated to the struggle for and preservation of civil rights for multiracial individuals and interracial couples/families." The site includes tons of links to multiracial magazines and sites.

The Natural Haven at http://thenaturalhaven.blogspot.com is the blog of a scientist who explains the science behind hair care and hair-care ingredients, with lots of juicy detail—and illustrations! This is a wonderful hair and ingredient resource, especially when you are looking for a deeper understanding of what's really in a product.

RACE at www.understandingrace.org. RACE works to destroy racial stereotypes. It explains scientifically why our skin evolved in different shades. It also helps promote understanding of the experiences of all kinds of people of different ages and races. There's even a link for kids to check out.

The Topaz Club at www.thetopazclub.com. The Topaz Club is a networking-support group of professional women with mixed African American ancestry. It has plenty of current information and links.

The World of Hair at www.pgbeautygroomingscience.com/the-world-of-hair1.html. This site by Dr. John Gray has a wealth of scientific information about the physiology and care of hair. He even has some great electron microscope photos of hair strands with varying degrees of damage. It's a great reference site.

References

Begoun, Paula. *Don't Go Shopping for Hair Care Products without Me*. Renton, WA: Beginning Press, 2005.

"Does Silicone Suffocate Hair?" The Beauty Brains, June 13, 2008. http://thebeautybrains.com/?s=silicones+suffocate&x=0&y=0.

Gorman, Jessica. "Chemistry of Colors and Curls—Chemicals in Dyes Damage Hair." *Science News*, August 25, 2001. http://findarticles.com/p/articles/mi_m1200/is_8_160/ai_78545498/pg_1.

Gray, John. *The World of Hair*. P&G Hair Research Center. 2003. Procter & Gamble. http://www.pgbeautygroomingscience.com/the-world-of-hair1.html.

Massey, Lorraine, with Deborah Chiel. *Curly Girl: More Than Just Hair—It's an Attitude: A Celebration of Curls: How to Cut them, Care for Them, Love Them, and Set Them Free*. New York: Workman, 2001.

Nissel, Angela. *Mixed: My Life in Black and White*. New York: Villard Books, 2006.

Peck, M. Scott. *The Road Less Traveled: A New Psychology of Love, Traditional Values and Spiritual Growth*. New York: Simon and Schuster, 1978.

Pomey-Rey, Danièle. "Hair and Psychology" in *The Science of Hair Care*. Charles Zviak, ed. New York: Marcel Dekker, 1986.

Quadflieg, Jutta Maria. *Fundamental Properties of African-American Hair.* Dissertation. Aachen: Rheinisch-Westfälischen Technischen Hochschule, 2003.

Ruetsch, S.B., et al. "Secondary Ion Mass Spectrometric Investigation of Penetration of Coconut and Mineral Oils into Human Hair Fibers: Relevance to Hair Damage." *Journal of Cosmetic Science* 52 (2001): 169–184.

Thibaut, Sebastien, et al. "Human Hair Keratin Network and Curvature." *International Journal of Dermatology* 46 (2007): 7–10.

"Two Natural Oils That Make Your Hair Shiny and Strong." The Beauty Brains, May 14, 2007. http://thebeautybrains.com/2007/05/14/two-natural-oils-that-make-your-hair-shiny-and-strong.

Wikipedia. "Hair." September 28, 2007, http://en.wikipedia.org/wiki/Hair.

Winter, Ruth, M.S. *A Consumer's Dictionary of Cosmetic Ingredients.* New York: Three Rivers Press, 2005.

Zviak, Charles, ed. *The Science of Hair Care.* New York: Marcel Dekker, 1986.

Photo Credits

Pages 1 (top), 5 (bottom), 6, 7, 8 (top left, top right, bottom), 10 (bottom), 11, 13, 14 (left, middle), 108, Ruth Sheldon; pp. 1 (bottom), 10 (top right), 17, 18 (bottom), 20, 31, 32, 51, 53, 61, 62, 68, 69, 74, 75, 76, 77, 80, 83, 84, 85, 86, 87, 88, 89, 90, 93, 94, 101, 102, 111, 115, 119, 120, 121, 128 (right), 129, 130, 168, 170, 171, 201, 202, 203, 222, 223, 224, 227, 228, 229, 230, 231, 233, 235, 236, 237, 238, 239, 240, 241, 242, 243, 244, 244, 245, 246, 248, 249, 250, 252, 253, Teri LaFlesh; p. 5 (top), Hanna Read; pp. 8 (top middle), 10 (top left), 12, 15, Betty Crowe; p. 14 (right), David Brewster; pp. 18 (top), 175, Billy Read; p. 104, Aja Robinson; p. 105, Frances Glen; p. 106, Vanessa Drakeford; p. 107, Amber Osborne; p. 128 (left), Jon Crump; pp. 144, 145, 146, 147, 148, 149, Jennifer Billingsley; p. 150, Jencie Simmons; pp. 172, 173, Bob Evans; p. 174, April Stuckey.

Index

Page numbers in italics refer to illustrations.